6th Edition

Scope and Standards of Practice for Professional Telehealth Nursing

Copyright © 2018
American Academy of Ambulatory Care Nursing (AAACN)
East Holly Avenue/Box 56, Pitman, NJ 08071-0056
800-AMB-NURS | FAX 856-589-7463 | aaacn@ajj.com | www.aaacn.org

ISBN: 978-1-940325-54-5

Printed in the United States of America

Suggested Citation
American Academy of Ambulatory Care Nursing. (2018). *Scope and standards of practice for professional telehealth nursing* (6th ed). T. Anglea, C. Murray, M. Mastal, & S. Clelland (Eds.). Pitman, NJ: American Academy of Ambulatory Care Nursing.

Publication Management by
Anthony J. Jannetti, Inc., East Holly Avenue/Box 56, Pitman, New Jersey 08071-0056
Phone: 856-256-2300 | Fax: 856-589-7463 | www.ajj.com

Scope and Standards Revision Team

Co-Chairs and Co-Editors

Tabitha Anglea, MSN, RN, CCRN-K, LNC
Clinical Manager, National Contact Center Management
Hospital Corporation of America (HCA)
Madison, TN

Cynthia L. Murray, BN, RN-BC
Ambulatory Care Nurse Manager Clinical Operations
Veterans Health Administration (VHA)
Veterans Integrated Service Network (VISN) 4
Southern New Jersey and Delaware Health System

Advisors and Co-Editors

Debra L. Cox, MS, RN, CENP
AAACN Past President
Nurse Administrator, Connected Care
Mayo Clinic
Rochester, MN

Margaret F. Mastal, PhD, MSN, RN
AAACN Past President
Retired
Alexandria, VA

Co-Editor

Susan Clelland, MSN, RN
Nurse Manager, Ambulatory Care
Henry Ford Health System
Detroit, MI

Board Liaison

Rocquel Crawley, DHA, MBA, BSN, RNC-OB, NEA-BC
Director of Nursing & Operations, Ambulatory Care
VCU Medical Center
Richmond, VA

Standards Revision Task Force

Katherine K. Andersen, MSN, RN-BC, CCM
Care Manager, Boise Telehealth Hub
Veterans Health Administration (VHA)
Virtual-Integrated Multisite Patient Aligned Care Team
    (V-IMPACT)
Boise, ID

Valeri Batara Aymami, MSN, RN, CNS, PCNS-BC, CPN
Advance Practice Nurse/Clinical Nurse Specialist, Ambulatory
Services
Children's Hospital Colorado
Aurora, CO

Robert Doheny
LTJG/Operational Medicine Division Officer
United States Navy
Virginia Beach, VA

Susanna M. Gadsby, MSNc, MBA, RN, ONC
Clinical Nurse Educator, Ambulatory Care
Dartmouth Hitchcock Health System
Lebanon, NH

Sandra C. Gallarno, BSN, RN
Lead Care Coordinator - Telehealth
Home Telehealth Master Preceptor
Veterans Health Administration
Aleda E. Lutz Veterans' Administration Medical Center (VAMC)
Saginaw, MI

Christine M. Griffel, MSN, RN-BC
Registered Nurse Care Manager
Veterans Health Administration
Veterans Integrated Service Network (VISN) 4
Pittsburgh Healthcare System
Pittsburgh, PA

Kathy Kesner, MS, RN, CNS
Manager
UC Health
Denver, CO

Kimberly Marshall, MSN, RN
Registered Nurse Care Coordinator
Veterans Health Administration
Veterans Integrated Service Network (VISN) 7
Southeast Network
Myrtle Beach, SC

Maureen T. Power, MPH, RN, LNCC
Senior Nurse Consultant
Power & Cronin, LTD
Oak Brook, IL

Carol Rutenberg, MNSc, RN-BC, C-TNP
Telephone Triage Consulting, Inc.
Hot Springs, AR

Kathryn B. Scheidt, MSN, MS, RN
Senior Account Executive
AxisPoint Health
Westminster, CO

Ms. Sharon Steingass, MSN, RN, AOCN
Director, Nursing Innovation
OSU Wexner Medical Center - James Cancer Hospital
Columbus, OH

Collaborators

Care Coordination Transition Management and Ambulatory
Care Scope and Standard of Practice for Professional Nurses
Task Force
Chair Cynthia Murray, BN, RN-BC

RN Role Position Paper Update Task Force
Chair Susan Paschke, MSN, RN-BC, NEA-BC

Telehealth Task Force
Chair Suzanne N. Wells, MSN, RN

Scope and Standards Revision Team

Contributors

Mary Mescher Benbenek, PhD, APRN, CPNP, CFNP
Clinical Associate Professor
FNP Program Coordinator
University of Minnesota School of Nursing
Minneapolis, MN

Jill M. Berg, PhD, RN, FAHA, FAAN, ATA Telehealth SIG
Vice President of Education
Ascension Wisconsin
President and Dean
Columbia College of Nursing

Troy Garland, MBA, BA, RN
CNO & Vice President Clinical Innovation
Sensely

M. Elizabeth Greenberg, PhD, RN-BC, C-TNP, CNE
President, AAACN

Dan Nagel, PhD, RN
Assistant Professor Department of Nursing & Health Sciences
University of New Brunswick
Saint John, Canada

Mary Steffes, DNP, APRN, CNS
Clinical Assistant Professor
University of Minnesota School of Nursing
Minneapolis, MN

David Stewart, MHM, BNRN
Associate Director
Nursing and Health Policy
International Council of Nurses

James Robert Torok, LSW-MSW
Virtual Care Program Manager
Veterans Health Administration (VHA)
Veterans Integrated Service Network (VISN) 4
Grove City, PA

Reviewers

Eleanor M. Chapital, MSN RN-BC
Program Manager, Transition and Care Management Program
Southeast Louisiana Veterans Health Care System
New Orleans, LA

Nancy Elliott, DNP, MSN/Ed, RN
Home Telehealth
Veterans Health Administration (VHA)
Veterans Integrated Service Network (VISN) 4
Southern New Jersey and Delaware Health System

Lori J. Hill, BSN, RN, MS
Director of Professional Development, Ambulatory
Kaiser Permanente
Portland, OR

Amber Lynn Lamoreaux, MSN, BSN, RN, OCN®
Care Coordinator RN
Moffitt Cancer Center
Tampa, FL

Jessica Miller, BSN, RN
Gundersen Health System
Program Manager - Telemedicine
La Crosse, WI

Elaine E. Nestell, RN, ADN, BSHCA, MSHCA
Spinal Cord Virtual Care Coordinator
VA Puget Sound Health Care Center
Seattle, WA

Susan M. Paschke, MSN, RN-BC, NEA-BC
Adjunct Professor
Kent State University
Kent, OH

CAPT Andrea Petrovanie, MSN, RN-BC, CNS
Senior Nurse Officer
Naval Medical Center San Diego
San Diego, CA

Maureen Phillips, BSN, RN, PHN
Poison Information Specialist (retired)
Descanso, CA

Jane M. Quist, BSN, RNC-TNP
Advice Nurse
Kaiser Permanente
San Jose, CA

Mary Smith, MSN, RN-BC, C-EFM, CCE
Clinical Nurse Educator, Ambulatory Division
Center for Nursing Professional Practice and Research
The University of Chicago Medicine
Chicago, IL

David Stewart, MHM, BNRN
Associate Director
Nursing and Health Policy
International Council of Nurses

Mary Jo Vetter, DNP, RN, AGPCNP-BC
Director DNP Program
New York University, Rory Meyers College of Nursing
New York, NY

Contents

Introduction

The American Academy of Ambulatory Care Nursing (AAACN) is the professional nursing organization for registered nurses (RNs) practicing in ambulatory, telehealth, and other health care settings. As such, AAACN is responsible for establishing, maintaining, and publishing the scope and standards of professional ambulatory care and telehealth nursing practice. AAACN published the first edition of professional standards for ambulatory care RNs in 1987. Since then, revisions and updates have occurred on a regular basis as the health care environment evolved, evoking changes and expansions to the practice of nursing.

In 1997, AAACN officially embraced telephone nursing as a subspecialty of ambulatory care nursing and published the first edition of telephone nursing practice standards. In 2001, updated telehealth standards were published as *Telehealth Nursing Administration and Practice Standards.* In 2011, the revisions and updates were entitled, *Scope and Standards of Practice for Professional Telehealth Nursing.*

Expanding interests in the 2nd decade of the 21st century, AAACN embarked on a multi-year journey to develop the role of the ambulatory care RN in care coordination and transition management (CCTM). The journey included the development of a CCTM Model and Core Curriculum (AAACN, 2016) online courses and the publication of CCTM scope and standards of care.

As a result of AAACN's extended activities, the current AAACN published standards include:

- *Scope and Standards of Practice for RNs in Care Coordination and Transition Management* (2016)
- *Scope and Standards of Practice for Professional Ambulatory Care Nursing* (2017)
- *Scope and Standards of Practice for Professional Telehealth Nursing* (2018)

This 6th edition publication provides revisions to the *Scope and Standards of Practice for Professional Telehealth Nursing* (2011). It aligns telehealth nursing with extensive health care environmental and technological transformations. In the past couple of years, along with radical changes to the organizational systems providing care for persons in all types of health care settings, extensive new technology has emerged for providing telehealth services. These technologies include the Internet, computers, digital environment and tools, and telemonitoring equipment utilized in a virtual environment.

Telehealth is an umbrella term used to describe the wide range of health services delivered using telehealth technology across distances by all health-related disciplines. It includes the delivery, management, and coordination of health services that integrate electronic information and telecommunication technologies to expand access, improve outcomes, and eliminate unnecessary costs (Greenberg, Espensen, Becker, & Cartwright, 2003; Nagel & Penner, 2016). Telehealth activities focus on communicating and partnering with patients and/or other health professionals using telehealth technology across distant and diverse environments. These environments include ambulatory care, acute care, post-acute care, long-term care, home health care, educational conferences, and a wide variety of agencies in community settings.

This publication may be used by health systems to:

1. Develop the structures and processes of the delivery of telehealth nursing (e.g., policies, procedures, role descriptions, and competencies).

2. Govern the delivery of quality health care for patients, populations, and communities using telehealth practices and technology.

3. Expand and advance professional telehealth nursing knowledge, skills, and attitudes.

4. Expedite the development of care delivery process models of telehealth nursing that assure patient safety, delivery of quality care, ethical practice, and patient advocacy.

5. Evaluate professional telehealth nursing performance using performance appraisals, peer reviews, and reflective practice.

6. Stimulate participation in telehealth research and evidence-based practice.

7. Conduct quality assurance and performance improvement initiatives in clinical and organizational telehealth environments.

8. Advance professional telehealth nursing practices that improve patient health and the performance outcomes of health care institutions.

Overview: Scope and Standards of Practice for Professional Telehealth Nursing

This document, *Scope and Standards of Professional Practice for Telehealth Nursing* (6th edition), is an advancement of AAACN's body of work. The Scope presents new thinking about telehealth as an integral component of today's professional health care practice. New telehealth technologies have evolved different care delivery practices focusing on persons living in remote areas as well as those who cannot easily access clinical settings, as well as those seeking convenient alternate models of health care. Registered nurses (RNs), in multiple roles, integrate the new telehealth technology and activities into their unique practice settings.

Inspired by the vision, values, and traditions of the past, this edition of the scope and standards of telehealth nursing reflects current professional norms, practices, and expectations, and recognizes the constantly evolving landscape of professional health systems. This set of revisions represents the work of task force members who conducted a broad scope of activities between March 2017 and January 2018. Task force members searched a broad base of telehealth and nursing literature for knowledge and scientific evidence as well as consulted with telehealth professionals in diverse telehealth settings. Additional input was obtained through review and recommendations by telehealth nursing experts.

This 6th edition contains significant revisions from previous versions. The Scope contains statements of the specific definition and defining characteristics of telehealth nursing in different practice settings across the continuum of care. It also integrates telehealth elements into the concept of environment in the AAACN conceptual framework. Additionally, it incorporates a historical overview of the evolution of telehealth nursing as the use of innovative technologies spurred unique practices.

Sixteen Standards are included in the publication. The first six standards address the six phases of the nursing process. The remaining ten standards address professional performance in telehealth practice.

Each standard contains a statement of expected professional behaviors and two types of measurement criteria that identify competent compliance with the standard. The first set of competency criteria address RNs integrating telehealth technology and services into professional practice. The second set of competency criteria focus on the proficiencies expected of the telehealth executive, manager, and/or administrator. These distinct competencies clarify and specify the expectations for the distinct domains of clinical and administrative telehealth practice in a variety of health care settings.

Scope of Practice for Professional Telehealth Nursing

The Scope of Practice statement describes who, what, where, when, why, and how of nursing practice. Each of these questions must be answered if we are to provide a complete picture of the dynamic and complex practice of nursing, its membership, and evolving boundaries (ANA, 2015a).

The Scope includes a definition of professional telehealth nursing services, an identification of the defining characteristics, a specification of the conceptual framework, a description of the practice environment, a discussion of the science and art of telehealth nursing service, an identification of the multiple telehealth roles in health care settings, and a discussion of the professional trends and issues.

I. Definition of Professional Telehealth Nursing

Professional telehealth nursing is a complex, multifaceted specialty that encompasses independent and collaborative practice during encounters that use telehealth technology in a virtual environment. The comprehensive practice of telehealth nursing is one built upon a broad knowledge base of nursing and health sciences, and applies clinical expertise rooted in the nursing process. RNs use evidence-based information across a variety of health care settings to achieve and ensure patient safety and quality of care while improving patient outcomes. Telehealth RNs promote optimal wellness, participate in the management of acute illness, assist the patient to manage effects of chronic disease and disability, provide care coordination during care transitions, and provide support in end-of-life care (AAACN, 2011).

RNs play a critical role in the delivery of telehealth services. The development of the art and science of telehealth nursing practice has improved and expanded coordination of health services, reduced patient risk, and contributed significantly to care management models (Paschke et al., 2017). The telehealth RN is accountable for providing nursing care in accordance with relevant federal requirements, state laws and nurse practice acts, regulatory standards, standards of professional ambulatory care nursing practice, other relevant professional standards, and organizational policies (AAACN, 2011; ANA, 2015a).

Telehealth is an umbrella term used to describe a wide range of services delivered in nontraditional modalities, across distances, by a variety of health-related disciplines. A list of interchangeable definitions is found in the Appendix. For purposes of this document, the definitions compiled vary. In areas where two definitions are listed, they are complementary to each other and are meant to provide the reader with a comprehensive overview of terminology in the ever-changing telehealth environment.

Defining Characteristics

A telehealth encounter currently has a variety of clinical applications such as episodic primary care, urgent care, inpatient care, chronic disease management, wellness coaching, medication management, and behavioral health. Characteristics of the telehealth encounter will vary on the setting and patient need. Telehealth encounters may:

- Involve real-time visits or remote patient monitoring that can be synchronous (real time) or asynchronous (time lag).
- Utilize a variety of technology platforms which include but are not limited to use of a telephone, mobile smart devices, kiosks, and/or web-based and digital platforms.
- Involve one or more health care providers and may consist of provider-to-patient or provider-to-provider encounters.
- Be a single encounter or in a series of encounters based on the reason for telehealth encounter and patient needs.
- Involve one or a group of patients.

The following knowledge, skills, and attitudes are recommended characteristics for a RN utilizing telehealth interventions across multiple practice settings. The telehealth RN will:

1. Use knowledge and skills based on principles of the biological, physical, behavioral, and social sciences.
2. Use the nursing process when interacting with a patient during a telehealth encounter.
3. Employ critical thinking and synthesis of objective and subjective data obtained during the assessment to identify priorities and care needs.
4. Recognize signs and symptoms of an emergency and readily identify how to best support patients/families in the management of the emergency.
5. Employ clinical judgment and available evidence to expedite a nursing diagnosis and disposition. Assume accountability for coordination of care, includ-

ing the use and delegation of telehealth activities to licensed practical nurses (LPNs) and unlicensed assistive personnel (UAP).

6. Deliver holistic patient-centered care, with the promotion of optimal health outcomes throughout the lifespan and across the health-illness continuum.

7. Demonstrate an appreciation of the environmental context that encompasses culture, ethics, law, politics, economics, and access to health care resources when interacting with the patient.

8. Act as an advocate to advise, assist, and support patients in the optimal management of their health care, respecting their individual needs, health goals, and treatment preferences.

9. Focus on patient safety and quality when applying appropriate nursing interventions.

10. Facilitate continuity of care using the nursing process, interprofessional collaboration, and coordination of appropriate health care services and community resources across the care continuum.

11. Demonstrate leadership knowledge and skills to support the clinical and administrative operations of the telehealth interventions across practice settings.

12. Design, administer, practice, and evaluate telehealth nursing services in accordance with relevant federal requirements, state laws, nurse practice acts, regulatory and accreditation standards, and institutional policies and procedures.

13. Apply the provisions of the ANA *Code of Ethics for Nurses* (ANA, 2015b) to their own professional practice.

14. Pursue lifelong learning and maintain competencies for telehealth nursing.

15. Participate in, contribute to, and/or apply research and evidence-based literature to improve the practice of telehealth nursing.

Objectives of Telehealth Nursing

The major objectives of telehealth nursing align with other types of nursing to:
- Protect and promote health.
- Minimize suffering.
- Maximize health literacy and education.
- Prevent illness and injury.
- Apply nursing interventions to human responses in health, illness, disease, disability, and end-of-life circumstances.
- Actively advocate for optimal coordinated health care of individuals, families, communities, and populations aimed at improving the whole person's well-being.

Interactions between patients and telehealth RNs to achieve patient goals occur in the context of caring, compassion, and sensitivity to the patient's cultural, ethnic, and age-related needs. The RN utilizes telehealth tools and the nursing process to deliver care in a variety of nursing roles and practice settings across distances.

II. Conceptual Framework

The Ambulatory Care Nursing Conceptual Framework can be used to describe the role of the RN working in a telehealth environment. The conceptual framework for ambulatory care nursing identifies three major concepts and the links between and among them: patient, nurse, and environment.

Patient

Inherent within the concept of patient is that each individual is unique; functions holistically as a biological, psychosocial, spiritual being; and is the center of nurse-patient interactions. In the health care setting, the nurse may not only interact with the patient but may also include interactions with family members, caregivers, support systems, groups, and populations that may be actively involved in the patient's care. Patient health states are categorized as wellness or health, acute illness, chronic disease, disability, and end-of-life care.

Contact or interaction can be initiated by the patient or nurse and the frequency and method of interaction is dependent on the patient's status, disease, and disability. Patients are always the central focus and maintain control of the encounter and treatment with the nurse in a consultative role.

Nurse

Telehealth nursing is an integral component of professional ambulatory care nursing practice that focuses on individuals, families, groups, communities, and populations in primary, specialty care, non-acute community outpatient settings, and in virtual environments. The scope of professional nursing is dynamic, responding to changing societal, organizational, and technological events as well as to the expanding knowledge base of nursing's theoretical and scientific domains (ANA, 2015a).

The telehealth RN component originally evolved when professional nurses were available to patients by telephone to ensure increased access to health care. The nurses triaged the patient to appropriate levels of care. Telehealth nursing has now expanded to include the delivery of more sophisticated nursing care, using various kinds of telehealth technology across distances in multiple types of virtual environments.

Professional RNs have three major role dimensions: professional, clinical, and organizational/systems. While defined separately, these role dimensions are not necessarily mutually exclusive and frequently overlap. The overlap of these role dimensions brings challenges and professional growth, adding dynamism, learning, and diversity in professional nursing practice.

Professional nursing role. The professional RN practicing in a telehealth role functions according to professional, ethical, governmental/regulatory, and organizational standards. As a practice expectation, the professional RN exhibits leadership skills within the health care organization, in the greater community, and across the nursing profession.

Professional practice requires the use of evidence-based scientific knowledge, measurement and evaluation of outcomes, and personal lifelong expansion of nursing knowledge and skills. The professional RN using telehealth technologies contributes to the knowledge and skills of other staff, health care providers, and is actively committed to continuous improvement of health care practices and outcomes.

Clinical nursing role. Professional RNs using telehealth technology regardless of their specialty or setting, practice using the nursing process and evidence-based nursing knowledge to guide interactions. Nurses in all care settings including telehealth require a broad array of competencies:

1. Use of evidence-based resources, protocols, and decision support tools.

2. Competent nursing process skills.

3. Ability to manage acute responsive episodes of care as well as proactive, recurrent scheduled encounters for health promotion and prevention.

4. Ability to critically analyze, integrate, and synthesize subjective and objective data related to patient concerns and conditions into the context of the patient's health situation and living environment.

5. Identifying and prioritizing pertinent problems and goals.

6. Creating and implementing nursing care interventions.

7. Evaluating the effectiveness of care provided.

8. Use technologies required to complete the telehealth encounter.

Additionally, the clinical role encompasses patient advocacy, referring patients to optimal health services within the organization and across the care continuum, health promotion and disease prevention education, and mediating secondary complications. In some cases, the nurse's role is to help the patient understand the trajectory of disease and to help him/her to plan for, adapt to, and manage his/her needs as health status changes.

This clinical role may include performing appropriate independent nursing interventions, consulting and collaborating with professional colleagues for their unique expertise for interdependent care, and functioning as part of an interprofessional team to implement a shared plan to achieve optimal patient outcomes. Professional telehealth RNs maintain accurate and timely documentation of care, and keep other members of the care team informed of changes in patient condition and/or the plan of care.

Organizational and/or systems role. Professional RNs functioning in the systems role administer and coordinate resources, and direct clinical workflow and ac-

tivity within their health care environments. The organizational role also includes collaboration with other health care professionals, resources, and agencies across the care continuum.

This role has multiple dimensions: leadership, staffing, workload, and competency concerns; workplace regulatory compliance and risk management; fiscal management; legal and regulatory issues; organizational cultural competence; and application of health informatics applications. It also includes diagnostic and treatment technologies, systems, research, and health advocacy within the organization and across the care continuum.

While some functions of all three roles are part of every RN's practice, emphasis on one of the roles usually exists depending on the specific functional position of the nurse within the practice setting. For example, whether functioning in face-to-face or virtual encounters, nurses will most likely focus on the clinical role requirements of their job description. However, organizational and professional role requirements may be expected concurrently depending on the organization's structure and the unique situation.

Environment

Environment as a concept continues to define ambulatory care and telehealth nursing practice. Recent changes in the health care landscape confirm environment is increasingly important to other nursing specialties. In addition to unique nurse-patient relationships and interactions, ambulatory care and telehealth nurses address organizational, social, economic, legal, and political factors within the health care system, the external health care environment, and in virtual environments. A virtual environment is defined as an environment other than the one in which the participants are physically present (Nagel, 2014; Wilson, 1997). Conceptually, environment has two major dimensions: internal and external.

Internal care delivery environment. The professional nursing practice delivery environment is dynamic and diverse. Within the internal environment there is interaction between patient and nurse. This interaction occurs either as a face-to-face or as a virtual encounter. Ambulatory care nursing and telehealth nursing may include a broad scope of multifaceted practice settings where patients seek health care treatment and where the professional RN functions. The use of virtual encounters in a telehealth setting provides the opportunity to provide care across distances.

External health care environment. The external environment refers to the physical location of each health care practice and includes other health care settings. Additionally, the external environment includes social determinants of health and health resource agencies across the greater environment that affect professional nursing practice.

The external geographical locale, available health care resources, and social determinants of health often influence that setting's mission, patient population, and practices. These external factors include other health

Figure 1.
Ambulatory Care Nursing Conceptual Framework Diagram

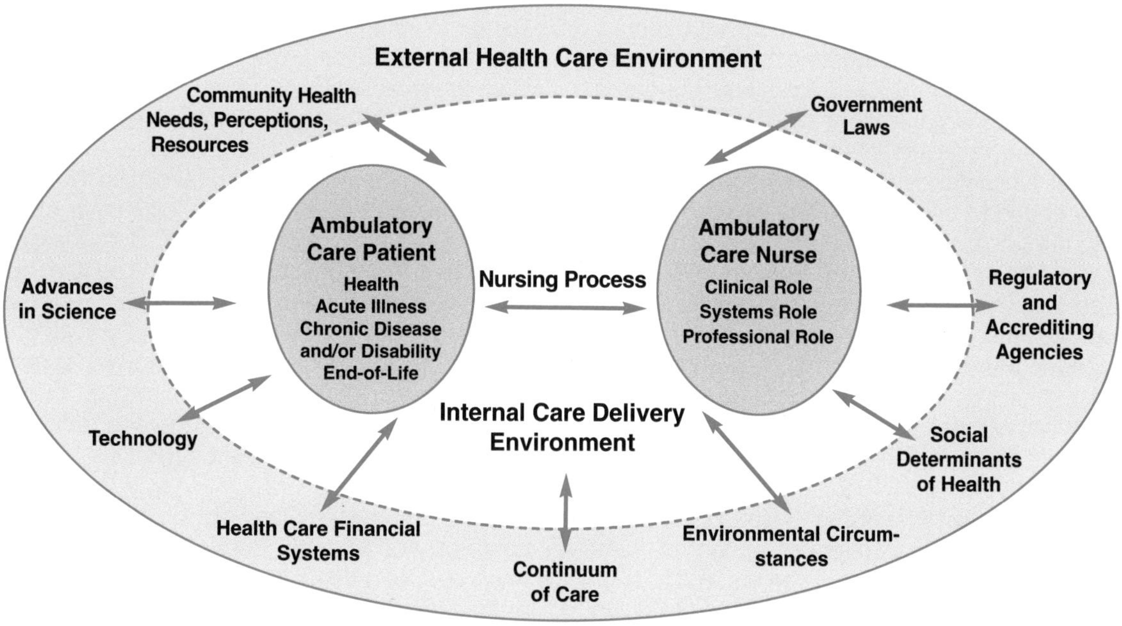

Source: Copyright © 2018. American Academy of Ambulatory Care Nursing

care settings, but are not necessarily limited to:

- Government laws (local, state, and/or federal).

- Regulatory, accrediting agencies, and professional practice regulations (Centers for Medicare & Medicaid Services, The Joint Commission, professional nursing organizations, etc.).

- Social determinants of health care which include socioeconomic status, education, physical environment, employment, social support network, and access to care (World Health Organization [WHO], 2017).

- Environmental circumstances (safety, transportation, pollution, disasters, epidemics, and/or pandemics, etc.).

- The extent and composition of the continuum of care.

- Health care financial systems (private insurers, Medicare, Medicaid, Veterans Health Administration, etc.).

- Types of technology (telehealth, information management, diagnostic, and treatment).

- Advances in science (scientific and evidence-based knowledge).

- The surrounding community population's specific needs, perceptions, and resources.

- The unique needs of the population served under population health programs (e.g., congestive heart failure, diabetes, mental health diagnoses, etc.).

Telehealth nursing is also present in other health care settings. An example would be post-discharge phone calls that occur from either the ambulatory care clinics or inpatient settings. Telehealth nursing practices in the inpatient settings may include eICU, tele-rounding, specialty nurse consultation by e-visits, and acute care monitoring. See Figure 1 for the conceptual diagram of telehealth nursing.

III. Evolution of Modern Telehealth Nursing Practice

Historically, telehealth was first introduced in the 19th century. However, it was during the 20th century that telehealth nursing emerged and expanded. Now, in the 21st century, telehealth in general and the practice of telehealth nursing has expanded exponentially due to development of innovative technologies, new legislative mandates, changes in health care reimbursement, and shortages of providers and RNs.

Early Origins: 19th Century

Telehealth as we know it today was first practiced by Alexander Graham Bell shortly after he invented the telephone in 1876. He spilled battery acid on himself and asked for help over the phone line (Darkins & Cary, 2000). In 1879, an article in *The Lancet* discussed using the telephone to reduce unnecessary office visits (Institute of Medicine [IOM], 2012). This was the first time delivery of health care over the telephone was documented in the literature. The telephone became key to delivering health care in the home, and not just in the provider's office.

20th Century: A Changing Healthcare Landscape

Legislative mandates changed the health care landscape in the 1970s and 1980s. Legislation endorsed Health Maintenance Organizations (HMOs) and established a capitated reimbursement system. Capitation failed to cover all health care expenses and it became clear costs needed to be reduced. The need to contain costs led to utilization of nurses in the role of patient interface with the health care system. These nurses, often called *triage* or *advice* nurses, helped patients determine the appropriate time, place, and manner to access care. Thus, telephone triage nurses became viewed as *gatekeepers*. In a system designed for cost containment, they directed patients to different levels of care, and were regarded by some as barriers to care (Rutenberg & Greenberg, 2012).

In the same general time frame, hospitals identified nurse-staffed call centers as effective public relations tools. The role of nurses in these call centers was to support marketing initiatives, such as health fairs, physician referrals, and provide health education and advice. With time, the role of telephone triage and advice nursing evolved within these hospital-based call centers as well as in HMOs, insurance companies, and other proprietary entities. Additionally, telephone triage and other forms of telehealth nursing were being practiced in most, if not all, ambulatory care settings, but its presence and significance were largely unrecognized (Rutenberg & Greenburg, 2012).

During the 1990s, it was recognized that telephone triage RNs provided new and valuable services, improved access to health care, and redirected patients to appropriate levels of care, generally facilitating positive clinical outcomes with more efficient use of resources (Rutenberg & Greenberg, 2012). Additionally, these RNs provided patient education, and increased physician, patient, and nurse satisfaction while providing cost-effective quality care (Omery, 2003).

As the practice of telephone triage became more robust, many nurses were practicing under the guidance and authority of largely physician-developed decision support tools and served to support the medical model of care. However, AAACN members recognized a need for a stronger professional identity and the organization established standards specific to telehealth nursing. AAACN also endorsed a national certification for Telephone Nursing Practice by the National Certification Corporation (NCC) from 2001-2007.

In 2007, it was decided that telehealth nursing was not a specialty or a sub-specialty, but rather an *integral component* of ambulatory care nursing (AAACN, 2007). It was recognized that a wide base of knowledge of ambulatory care nursing was essential to the successful practice of telehealth nursing. Further, knowledge of the practice of telehealth nursing and utilization of telecommunications technology should be part of the basic skill set for all ambulatory care nurses (C. Rutenberg, personal communication, August 14, 2017). Subsequently, AAACN worked with the American Nurses Credentialing Center to incorporate telehealth content into the Ambulatory Care Nursing Certification Exam (Rutenberg & Greenberg, 2012).

21st Century Changes: Technology Explosion

Although the telephone was key to the practice of early and maturing telehealth nursing in the 20th century, innovative changes in technology have continued to move telehealth practice forward. Both the government and private entities have recognized the benefits of changes to improve disparities in health care in remote and rural settings. The invention and growth of the Internet and other technologies have allowed for rapid growth of telehealth. Telehealth promises to bring "untold change to the healthcare industry and radically improve the delivery of care to patients" (Darkins & Cary, 2000, p. 2).

The Affordable Care Act of 2010 funded patient-centered Accountable Care Organizations that created new roles for nursing in care coordination and transition management (Haas, Swan, & Haynes, 2014). These new roles rely heavily on telehealth technology. The increased incidence of chronic illness, rising health care costs, and increased emphasis on the delivery of quality care have influenced the development of services that incorporate telehealth nursing as a care delivery strategy that provides disease management, care management, case management, and clinical prevention services (AAACN, 2013).

Modern consumers have come to expect their care will be delivered conveniently and quickly via electronic means. Health care systems, in order to compete for dwindling resources, including providers and RNs, will continue to increase the use of telehealth technologies to deliver health care.

Nurses are involved in three main modalities of telehealth:

1. Real-time telehealth, also known as synchronous or live telehealth, uses interactive video technology in care, generally between a health care provider and a patient.

2. Asynchronous telehealth incorporates transmission of prerecorded information, such as photos or X-rays, to specialists for interpretation.

3. Remote patient monitoring utilizes electronic monitoring devices from home, community, or on patient's person to capture physiologic data and patient's symptoms. Nurses review the information and coordinate care as necessary (Darkins & Cary, 2014). Digital technologies will continue to grow and dominant future health care delivery.

Today, telehealth continues to reshape nursing practice across the health care continuum. Because of the need to decrease the spiraling costs of health care, increase access to care in community sites, support the growing numbers of aging and chronically ill patients, and to bring care to both urban and rural areas, telehealth nursing continues to expand. Telehealth nursing services are patient friendly, convenient, and facilitate ease of use for patients. Telehealth encounters decrease the distance and amount of travel required to access health care, decrease readmission to inpatient settings by enabling frequent monitoring of patient's health states, and supply nursing services in areas where shortages exist.

IV. Practice Environment: Virtual

With the increasing use of technology to support access to health care, there is an expanding role for nursing in the utilization and leadership in the use of telehealth technologies. "The importance of telehealth as a major vehicle for delivering timely care over distance has become increasingly relevant as the world's heath care needs have become overwhelmed by a significant increase in the global level of chronic disease" (Dinesen et al., 2016, para. 2). The Macy Foundation (2016) report indicates RNs can increase access to care by assisting with management of chronic disease, substance abuse, and mental health patients. The telehealth nurse can improve transitional care as patients move throughout the complex health care system.

Benefits of telehealth are well recognized and include increased access to health care, better health outcomes, and more cost-effective service delivery (Nagel et al., 2016). Telehealth provides the right care at the right time and in the right place. Patients are no longer required to travel long distances to attain optimal outcomes, nor are they limited to receiving needed services at fixed practice sites (Lipstein & Kellermann, 2016). Telehealth offers the opportunity to deliver patient-centered care that is both accessible and convenient, overcoming many of the barriers in traditional health care delivery systems (Dinesen et al., 2016). Telehealth encounters occur in clinic settings, on the telephone, or by electronic messaging, and in other non-face-to-face (virtual) environments that are convenient for the patient. Encounters are generally, although not always, initiated by the individual seeking information and/or care. This practice environment allows for the export of nursing expertise to patients and encompasses specific practice settings, usually defined in terms of the medical specialty, and resources of the institution(s). Understanding and defining organizational, provider, and patient access will determine the most effective operating environment. The RN can also improve consumer engagement, quality scores, and collaboration within the health care team.

Practice Settings

Telehealth care spans primary care (when the patient first seeks care) through acute care, chronic and disability care follow-up, and palliative care in end-of-life situations in a variety of settings such as hospital based, skilled nursing facility, and assisted living. Telehealth RNs care for patients in all phases of preventive care, health maintenance, diagnosis, treatment, and follow-up, as patients move across the health care continuum.

It is important for all health care providers to maintain a patient-centered approach to care. This care is focused on adapting to the virtual environment where the communication techniques allow for sound clinical assessments and preservation of safe clinical relationships at a distance (Guise & Wiig, 2017). Nursing must utilize sound clinical assessment skills and provide appropriate, safe, and holistic care in clinical practice; this remains imperative with the shift from traditional face-to-face encounters to a virtual environment where information exchange is digitally mediated (Nagel et al., 2016).

For nurses in the virtual environment, hearing the patient's story, extracting relative subjective and objective data, and formulating conclusions about the patient's needs are essential to the effective delivery of nursing care. The nurse must utilize highly effective communication skills to obtain sufficient and clear information for creating a mental image or "getting a picture" of a person.

The dimensions for getting a picture of the patient include:

- Entering in the relationship
- Connecting with the person
- Sharing and reviewing information
- Recognizing patterns and trends
- Recording and reflecting patient information
- Putting pieces together over time
- Transitioning out (Nagel et al., 2016)

Types of Telehealth Care Organizations

Telehealth nursing functions in a variety of health care organizations as part of an organized nursing department under a nurse executive with a voice at the governing body level. Advancements made by the Magnet® nursing status, Pathways to Excellence, and The Joint Commission, require nursing leadership authority over nursing practice. Some health care settings continue to have nurses reporting to non-nursing leadership that may impact the standard of nursing practice and delivery of nursing services.

Within the distinct types of health care settings there may also be internal differences based on size, regional location, network or health system affiliation, and regional differences in health finance administration.

Telehealth occurs in the following organizational settings:

- Care management or care coordination centers
- Ambulatory care settings
- Inpatient settings
- Government health systems, including military settings
- Telehealth service centers
- Urgent care centers or emergency departments

- Long-term care
- Schools
- Behavioral health facilities

The practice environment of nurses working in various telehealth roles is diverse and numerous and is intimately linked and integrated with the American health care system. See Figure 2 for the context of telehealth nursing practice as an integral component of ambulatory care nursing practice.

Treatment Episodes

The patient or health care provider originates an episode of care in the telehealth environment. Direct observation technology may not always be readily available in all cases. Thus, the nurse may have to rely on patient-reported symptoms. RNs use the nursing process during assessment and treatment episodes that are effective and/or patient/family centered and controlled. With telehealth encounters, the RN must offer encouragement and meaningful insight into patient data throughout the patient's progress or patient participation may decline (Dinesen et al., 2016).

Treatment plan. The management of the treatment plan in the telehealth setting is largely the responsibility of the patient/family system. The RN, as consultant and advocate, pursues a more comprehensive understand-ing of the patient's condition. Effectively questioning for additional subjective and objective data avoids gaps in critical information needed to make clinical judgments about diagnosis and care. Health care organizations continue to acquire more sophisticated information systems. Increasingly, RNs have access to more objective data regarding the patient's health status such as medical history, specialist visits, medications, and test results.

The telehealth environment has not only created change for the nurse but also for the consumer. This modality of care requires consumers to have a greater trust in themselves and their own ability to make lifestyle changes and carry out health-related actions. This trust in themselves was previously placed with their health care professionals. The health care professional has the new task of facilitating these changes for the consumer.

Care interventions. Historically, interventions by telehealth RNs tended to be patient initiated and focused on health care advice. RNs provided instructions on how to manage a condition in the home or how to prepare for diagnostic testing. In recent years, patients with more complex conditions and/or treatment regimens have received care from RNs in both inpatient and outpatient settings. In both settings, telehealth nursing continues to expand and evolve. Care interventions commonly applied by the telehealth nurse include:
- Identifying and clarifying patient needs.

Figure 2.
Context for Ambulatory Care Nursing Practice

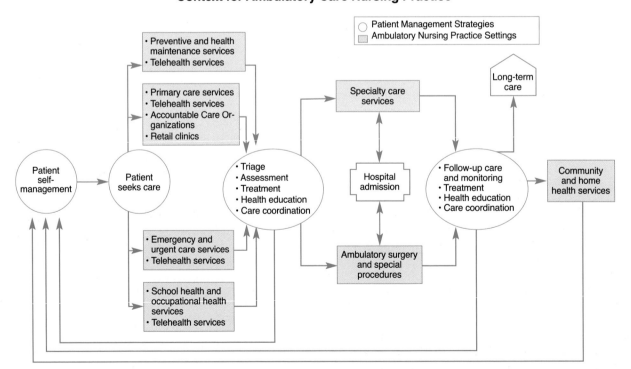

Source: Adapted from Hastings, 2013 and AAACN/ANA, 1997.

- Conducting health education.
- Promoting patient advocacy and self-efficacy.
- Coordinating nursing and other health services.
- Assisting the patient to navigate the health care system.
- Consulting and collaborating with other health care professionals.
- Facilitating the development of an intraprofessional care plan.
- Evaluating patient outcomes.

Nursing Workload: Variable

Telehealth nursing is as variable as the modalities through which it is delivered. Factors affecting workload include what is being monitored or assessed, the modality being utilized, and the frequency and duration. Available support services and requirements for electronic health record (EHR) documentation may also affect workload. It is important to have quality monitoring and improvement processes in place to assist with responding to changes in circumstances, assessing unexpected performance, and identifying improvements. The primary goal of telehealth is improved clinical outcomes alongside more efficient use of clinician time (Sharma & Clarke, 2014). Workload requirements and population needs can be researched by utilizing data contained in the EHR system; other workload management tools include call management systems.

V. The Science and Art of Telehealth Nursing Practice

Telehealth nursing practice is a learned practice requiring the application of a core body of knowledge from the biological, physical, behavioral, and social sciences. Telehealth nursing utilizes a variety of telecommunication technologies during encounters to assess, triage, provide nursing consultation, and perform follow-up and surveillance of patients' status, interventions, and outcomes (AAACN, 2013). Telehealth nursing is both an art and a science, combining professional knowledge with interpersonal and technical skills.

Science of Telehealth Nursing Practice

The science of telehealth nursing is based on a six-step nursing process: nursing assessment, diagnosis, goal/outcome identification, planning, implementation, and evaluation. These steps are central to the clinical decision-making process and are used in evidence-based practice.

Telehealth nursing focuses on needs of patients in all phases of health, illness, and disease, assisting patients to promote and maintain health and prevent or mediate illness, disease, or disability. The nursing needs of patients are assessed holistically, using available objective data as well as subjective data from the patient and family. In telehealth nursing, gathering data, especially objective data, requires the use of the art as well as the science of telehealth nursing. While nursing diagnosis and treatment(s) are similarly focused on the patient's goals, implementation and evaluation of progress toward outcomes are patient centered and patient driven and of a collaborative nature.

In addition, the use of decision support tools, if available, involves the use of science, supporting clinical judgment and decision-making process. The tools should be evidence based, using data and outcomes to drive the nursing process. Decision support tools suggest assessment parameters, and guide the nurse in collecting a relevant history and suggesting appropriate dispositions, education, and advice (Rutenberg & Greenberg, 2012).

Art of Telehealth Nursing Practice

The art of nursing practice applies to all telehealth nursing roles. It is based on respect for the dignity of others and compassionate caring, embracing a multitude of dynamic processes that affect human interaction. These dynamic processes are aspects that foster health and healing:

- Listening
- Assisting
- Mentoring
- Coaching
- Empathizing
- Teaching
- Exploring
- Providing presence
- Cultural competence
- Accepting
- Nurturing
- Resolving conflicts

In telehealth nursing, knowing the patient presents additional challenges. It is often a single interaction, and the interaction relies on remote technology to convey the intangible aspects of nursing. Telehealth nursing allows the opportunity to augment a nurse/patient relationship, taking the relationship beyond the clinic and acute care setting (Nagel, 2014).

Telehealth nurses employ practices that in nature are:

- **_Restorative:_** Practices that modify or mediate the clinical impact of illness, disease, or disability.
- **_Supportive:_** Practices that modify the impact of clinical/organizational/professional concern or dysfunction.
- **_Promotive:_** Practices that mobilize healthy patterns of living and quality of life for individuals, families, organizations, communities, and populations (ANA, 2004, p. 10).

Professional Responsibility

The practice of telehealth nurses is affected by the changing needs of society, the expanding knowledge base of nursing's theoretical and scientific domains, and growing health care technology. Nurses need to place themselves at the center of development, acting as a voice for their patients and profession. During an encounter, the RN focuses on patient safety and quality of nursing care by applying appropriate nursing interventions (AAACN, 2013) and using critical thinking during the nursing process.

Professional responsibility requires multiple and diverse skills:

• Visionary leadership in practice settings

• Inclusion of the community and the profession

• Management skills in patient care settings and profession

• Sound personal and professional ethical code

• Continual ambulatory nursing knowledge development

• Review and evaluation of nursing practice

• Evaluation of and improvement in the quality of patient and organizational outcomes

• Evaluation of safety

• Assessment of the effectiveness and costs in planning and delivering nursing care

• Maintenance of communication with the patient, family, and/or caregivers

For telehealth nursing, this means addressing the lack of pertinent research and potential for fragmented care. In addition, more research addressing telehealth nursing outcomes is needed, and the telehealth nurse should lead the way.

VI. Types of Telehealth Nursing Roles

The practice of telehealth nursing is the responsibility of the RN. Due to the complexity and potential for ambiguity associated with the provision of care via telehealth, it is essential that nursing care be managed by a licensed professional who is formally educated to exercise clinical judgment and utilize critical thinking. Telehealth nursing represents independent nursing practice in a highly collaborative environment (Rutenberg & Greenberg, 2012). Therefore, nurses undertaking telehealth roles must have the education and experience necessary to support critical thinking and complex decision making.

Nursing care delivery utilizing telehealth technology can be embodied in three distinct categories:

1. **Triage** or management of symptom-based encounters most often occurs over the telephone but may occur via videoconferencing or other types of telehealth technology. Due to the level of sophistication necessary for safe management of symptom-based calls, triage is performed exclusively by RNs. In telehealth triage, in which the nature and urgency of the call are unpredictable, RNs should be able to manage a full range of calls, from simple to complex. Novice nurses need specific support for role development and enhanced clinical expertise via structured competency-based programs.

2. **Coordination of Care and Transition Management** involves chronic care management, behavioral modification, and other patient care activities. Elements of the nursing process requiring critical thinking may not be delegated. The processes of care coordination and transition management (Coleman & Boult, 2003) necessitate professional assessment, patient risk identification and stratification, and identification of individual patient needs and preferences that require:

   a. Interprofessional collaboration and teamwork.
   b. Evidence-based care delivery.
   c. Patient and/or caregiver activation and empowerment.
   d. Utilization of quality and safety standards.
   e. Ability to work independently in the domain of nursing to identify and access community resources that meet individual, group, or population needs (AAACN, 2016).

3. **Remote Patient Monitoring** nursing roles include both short-term and longer-term acute and chronic care assessment and interventions with both patients and consumers. Nursing roles are focused on supporting adoption of self-care management techniques and increased health promotion and prevention behaviors. Nursing roles have evolved as technology and ability to share physiologic data is enhanced through technological advancements in wearables, sensors, and digital tools that impact both the timeliness and scope of data available to the RN and care team. New technologies are classified as either medical grade or consumer grade; each provide for enhanced patient data exchange which may challenge health care teams identifying appropriate, scalable, and meaningful interactions with patients and consumers. Clinical decision support, artificial intelligence, machine learning, and "big data" practices will provide opportunities to determine meaningful data sets and health care interventions for the future (Rigla, Garcéa-Sáez, Pons, & Hernando, 2017). Nurse-led traditional patient remote monitoring programs are well-accepted methods for supporting patients in managing their chronic care health issues. As technology advances, many new health care tools will support nurses in providing interactive nursing care for patients experiencing shorter-term needs such as post-hospitalizations, procedures, and clinic-based episodes of care. Health care will be provided through patient software applications such as interactive care plans on a smartphone, implantable as well as noninvasive monitoring technologies for specialty-specific acute and chronic needs, and short-term data monitoring to identify trends and patterns of health or disability

fueling predictive health analyses. Finally, nurses' "web-side" competence in use of video technology, utilization of digital data, and mastery of personalization of care will be critical skills to support emerging models of care which rely on technology as a foundation of interaction with patients.

Delegation to non-RNs

All encounters requiring assessment, nursing diagnosis, goal setting, planning, and/or evaluation must be conducted by an RN. Delegation to other staff may be appropriate within this category; however, any encounter that unexpectedly presents a symptom should be transferred to an RN for triage (Rutenberg & Greenberg, 2012).

To assure RNs work to the top of their license and to assure cost effectiveness (AAACN, 2017a, 2017b), some elements of telehealth nursing may be delegated to non-RNs. When elements of telehealth nursing tasks are delegated to LPN/LVNs or UAP, these individuals are functioning under the supervision of the RN or a provider.

VII. Professional Trends and Issues

The practice of telehealth nursing continues to evolve as the landscape of health care has shifted from a focus on acute illness to an emphasis on health and wellness in informed and empowered patients, families, and caregivers. Innovative telehealth practice settings provide solutions to the high incidence of chronic illnesses, shrinking health care resources, limited access to subspecialty providers, and an ever-expanding patient population. Among these challenges is the need to partner with and advocate for patients as they navigate through the complex and fragmented health care system. This shift in focus is accompanied by new initiatives such as care coordination and transition management across the care continuum, health promotion and disease prevention, and emphasis on population health and wellness across the lifespan. Customer satisfaction and measurable outcomes are critical indicators of quality care delivery. A new generation of innovative technology is providing patient-centric solutions.

Telehealth nursing is an important outgrowth of this movement. Instead of a primary focus on delivery of care in the face-to-face setting (in either acute or ambulatory care venues), the emphasis is now on learning new techniques to connect across distances with patients and their families or caregivers in their own environment. While the telephone continues to be a vital tool with which telehealth nursing care is delivered, nurses are utilizing other telehealth applications and technologies. Decision support tools are a foundational component of telehealth technologies. The evolution of machine learning and artificial intelligence is becoming more prevalent in health care and will also impact telehealth technology and nursing care. It is important to recognize that telehealth nursing is nursing provided via the use of telehealth technology rather than defined by the technology itself.

Enhanced Nurse Licensure Compact (eNLC)

In the mid to late 1990s, as telehealth nursing gained more visibility, the question of interstate practice became an issue. In 1997, the National Council of State Boards of Nursing (NCSBN) published *Position Paper on Telehealth Nursing Practice* in which they asserted nursing care delivered over distance using telecommunications technology is indeed the practice of nursing and is thus regulated by state boards of nursing (BONs) (NCSBN, 2014). Later, the NCSBN, along with the Federation of State Medical Boards and the National Association of Boards of Pharmacy, published a collaborative position statement declaring the locus of responsibility for a telehealth nursing encounter is at the location of the patient, family, and/or caregiver (Tri-Regulator Position Statement). Thus, nurses are practicing in the state in which the patient is located, regardless of the location of the nurse (NCSBN, 2014), even if the patient is only in the remote state temporarily (Rutenberg & Greenberg, 2012).

To address this regulatory concern, the Nurse Licensure Compact (NLC) was proposed in 1998. However, progress was stalled as only half the states passed legislation to join the Compact. In 2015, an eNLC was proposed to bring more states to the table. The theme of this revised compact is "Unlocking Access to Nursing Care Across the Nation" (NCSBN, 2017). Within about 2 years of development of the eNLC, the number of states in the Compact grew, with the opportunity for more states to be included.

Until uniform adoption of the eNLC is achieved, those practicing telehealth nursing remotely in non-Compact states will often continue to be at risk by either providing care across state lines, effectively practicing in remote states without a license, or declining to provide care to patients who seek their counsel. Short of each state enacting the eNLC, nurses in non-Compact states often find themselves in the difficult position of problem solving how best to assist callers when Compact state or licensure are in question. Technological solutions such as geo-caching assists organizations with matching licensed nurses by corresponding eNLC states to the patient's physical location. AAACN has supported the adoption of the eNLC to support telehealth nursing practice across state lines providing care regardless of where the patient is located.

Staffing and Role Confusion

Role confusion continues to exist in health care especially as it pertains to telehealth nurses practicing at the top of their license (IOM, 2012). Professional nursing needs to evaluate the scope of practice of the intended telehealth activities to assure appropriateness of staffing. Non-licensed staff may provide support to telehealth activities if RN assessment and judgment are not required. For example, some tele-presenting, telephonic communication, and secure messaging may be supplemented by non-licensed individuals. Telehealth encounters requiring critical thinking, clinical reasoning, and nursing judgment must be conducted by RNs regardless of the health care setting.

Medication Management

Another challenge in the telehealth setting involves the recommendation of medications. Boards of nursing and pharmacy vary in their positions and opinions regarding whether it is within the scope of practice for the RN to recommend over-the-counter (OTC) or prescription medications and under what circumstances. Some BONs regard recommendation of OTC medications as being within the independent scope of practice of the RN, other states will allow this action only based on a medically approved protocol, and others will not permit RNs to recommend OTCs under any circumstances. Recommendation or renewal of prescription medications is universally regarded as being outside the independent scope of practice of the RN. However, some states will allow RNs to initiate prescription medications or renew existing prescriptions using a medically approved protocol (Rutenberg & Greenberg, 2012).

Interprofessional Relationships

The relationship between the telehealth nurse and other members of the health care team is often misunderstood by members of both the nursing and the medical professions. Telehealth nursing, while collaborative, is independent nursing practice. The misconception that the nurse functions as an agent of the provider, with the provider being responsible for decision making, overlooks the significance of the nurse/patient relationship and fails to recognize the autonomy and responsibility held by the RN. Nurses play a critical role in the evolution of team-based care. Collaboration with other health care providers in the telehealth setting is evolving into a true partnership.

Telehealth Technology

Electronic/virtual visits, patient portals, and mobile device applications have joined structured telephone support and remote biophysical monitoring as tools in the nurse's toolkit. These tools enhance the ability to improve patient, family, and/or caregiver engagement in care, provide real-time health monitoring, lend support for patient self-management, and enhance communication between the patient and health care professionals. A growing body of evidence supports positive outcomes associated with many technologically enhanced interventions that provide health information and advice, support lifestyle modification, encourage medication adherence, enhance chronic condition management, and reduce unnecessary utilization (DeBlois & Millefoglie, 2015: Flodgren, Rachas, Farmer, Inzitari, & Shepperd, 2015; Vinson, McCallum, Thornlow, & Champagne, 2011; While & Dewsbury, 2011). Telehealth, technology is applicable in the following situations:

- Symptom triage and management
- Education and coaching
- Chronic care management
- Care coordination and transition management
- Patient, family, and/or caregiver activation
- Medication and treatment plans under protocols
- Transmission of diagnostic results
- Physiologic monitoring of patients
- Scheduling of appointments and referrals
- Other necessary health care functions

Electronic Health Records: The ability of health systems to support and coordinate patient care through virtual information exchange remains a priority in health care. For telehealth technology to be useful, it must be integrated, accessible, and user-friendly. To improve patient safety, a national incentive program to use electronic health records (EHRs) was offered through the American Recovery and Reinvestment Act of 2009). Implementation of EHRs has changed the way telehealth RNs practice and affected how services are provided in population health, transitions of care, and integrated care across the continuum of care.

Technological Challenges: Challenges remain in that not all telehealth nurses have access to the same type of technology, applications, and tools, nor are they always included in development of information technology applications. Education to support digital literacy in the health care setting is often lacking for nurses (ANA, 2015a). Federal and state regulation and funding is another major influence on the development and diffusion of telehealth technologies supporting innovative models of care.

These challenges impact the ability to streamline communication across the continuum of care and negatively impact efficiency. These inefficiencies can be measured in decreased customer and staff satisfaction, poor patient outcomes, and increased risk. An organization's ability to continually identify gaps in delivery of services and expand quality oversight will ensure improved processes for the telehealth nurse.

Shifts in Workplace: Advancing technologies have enabled the telehealth nurse to work virtually from remote locations. This shift in the defined workplace poses both advantages and challenges for the nurse and organization. Foremost among these challenges, as in all telehealth settings, is protection of patient privacy. Encryption of medical records is necessary, and patient privacy is maintained under government regulation and oversight.

Defining Quality Care and Outcomes

Societal, economic, and regulatory influences have moved health care in the United States toward reimbursement based on quality indicators. Quality of care and performance improvement have increased in visibility and intensity in the provision of telehealth services. The identification and definition of quality outcomes have been elusive in telehealth nursing. In the past, productivity measurements such as call length have been utilized to define and assess quality care. Now qualitative measures are emphasized with focus on structure, process, and outcome. Clinically oriented outcome measures are critical to the future of healthier patients and high-performing organizations (U.S. Department of Health and Human Services, 2018). Although quality care and patient safety are the primary goals of nursing practice, factors beyond the RN's control may impact the ultimate outcome for the patient. The identification and definition of clinical outcomes must focus on the telehealth encounter itself and include examination of the patient's engagement and ability to carry out the collaboratively developed plan of care.

Development of Nurse-Sensitive Indicators. AAACN has been invested in leading the way toward identification and development of ambulatory care nurse-sensitive indicators (NSIs). In 2013, AAACN commissioned a taskforce to identify and develop NSIs. By 2016 this taskforce proposed 13 indicator areas for further refinement, pilot testing, and eventual benchmarking (Mastal, Matlock, & Start, 2016). This important report was followed by the initiation of a partnership between AAACN and Collaborative Alliance for Nursing Outcomes (CALNOC). CALNOC, one of the original six pilot studies to develop inpatient indicators in the 1990s, was the scientific partner needed to guide AAACN clinical expertise into meaningful measurement for ambulatory settings.

The AAACN/CALNOC team expanded its partnership through continued work on NSI development that include indicators of the vital role nurses assume in telehealth, tele-triage, care coordination, transitions management, and other methods of virtual health care. These activities are crucial for access to care, reduction of acute care utilization, and promotion of health. Health care systems will benefit from NSI measurement that captures the important contributions of telehealth nursing.

Future Trends

As telehealth continues to expand and break down geographical barriers to care, improving efficiencies and access, identification of measures of care will be established. The U.S. Department of Health and Human Services called upon the National Quality Forum (2017) to convene a multi-stakeholder telehealth committee to recommend various indicators to measure use of telehealth as a means of providing care.

To maintain focus on patient care, provider organizations and telehealth RNs need to partner with and thus influence the diverse regulatory and accrediting agencies that set measurement standards for quality care. Quality, risk, and legal aspects are closely connected and continue to be a growing concern in telehealth nursing.

Undergraduate and Continuing Education

The basic skill set of telehealth nursing is not commonly addressed in undergraduate education. Many graduate nurses obtain basic education on telehealth nursing during their initial clinical orientation or nurse residency program (AAACN, 2017a, 2017b). However, ambulatory care and telehealth nursing standards are influencing many undergraduate clinical assignments within the curricula of baccalaureate-level nursing programs.

Telehealth nurses, just as all nurses, deal with continual changes in technology. This growth in technology and further development of telehealth nursing leads to the need for continuing education for the telehealth nurse. Currently, each agency and/or organization creates its own orientation and education program. Each nurse has an obligation to continuously maintain and update knowledge and competency as a lifelong learner (ANA, 2015a, 2015b). The telehealth nurse must regularly evaluate the impact of new knowledge and change on the scope of telehealth nursing practice, keeping in mind ethical and legal implications for the patient, nurse, and organization.

Summary

Over the past decade, health care has expanded its boundaries, a result of changing legislation, evolving reimbursement practices, and new technology. This new technology has improved the diagnosis and treatment of illness and disease, enlarged the practice of health care delivery, especially the practice of telehealth nursing, as well as developed new communication modalities among interprofessional providers, patients, caregivers, and resources across the health care continuum.

Related most importantly to telehealth nursing, the changes have expanded the definition of telehealth nursing and its defining characteristics, integrated new factors within the concept of the external environment in the conceptual framework, and developed new nursing roles in care coordination and transition management.

This document also explores the evolution and history of telehealth nursing, identifies current types of telehealth care organizations, and examines issues emanating from changes in the landscape of health care that affect nurses and other professionals in the telehealth environment. Discussion of gaps in education for telehealth practice are identified and recommendations made to close the gaps, so nurses are prepared to work to the top of their license. Finally, recommendations are offered for telehealth professionals to partner with government and regulatory agencies to set measurement standards for quality care, risk avoidance, and adherence to legal requirements. The standards that follow provide the details of the practice of nursing in the telehealth environment.

Standards of Practice for Professional Telehealth Nursing

The American Academy of Ambulatory Care Nursing (AAACN), as the specialty nursing organization for nurses practicing in ambulatory care, is responsible for establishing and publishing the standards for telehealth nursing practice. These standards are authoritative statements that describe the responsibilities for which telehealth nurses are accountable. In this version, the standards have been separated into two domains: *Clinical Practice* and *Professional Performance.*

Standards of Professional Clinical Practice

The six Clinical Practice Standards address the science and art of nursing clinical practice in ambulatory care – the nursing process. The nursing process is a rational, systematic method of planning and providing nursing care. It was developed by Ida J. Orlando in the late 1950s as she observed nurses as they practiced.

It has been refined by the profession over the intervening decades and now has six steps, applicable to both individuals and populations that are the basis of the standards of clinical practice in nursing (ANA, 2012).

- *Assessment:* The professional nurse's systematic, dynamic collection and analysis of the patient, group, and/or the population with the presenting concern, using physiological, psycho-socio-cultural, spiritual, economic, and lifestyle data as well as the patient's response to the problem.

- *Nursing Diagnosis:* Professional nursing statement that represents the nurse's clinical judgment about the patient's response to actual or potential health conditions or needs.

- *Identification of Expected Outcomes/Goals:* Professional nurse identifies, using input from the patient/family, other health professionals, and current scientific evidence, expected outcomes of an individualized plan of therapies and/or treatment(s).

- *Planning:* Professional nurse outlines a set of written statements that set measurable and achievable short and long-term goals to meet expected outcomes.

- *Implementation:* Professional nurse provides nursing care services to meet patient's needs and goals and documents all activities. Implementation involves a variety of roles:
  - Care Coordination/Transition Management
  - Health Teaching and Health Promotion
  - Consultation

- *Evaluation:* Professional nurse's continual appraisal of patient's status and effectiveness of care received, revising the care plan and interventions as appropriate.

Standards of Nursing Organizational and Professional Performance

The ten professional performance standards for telehealth nursing identify a competent level of behavior in the organizational and professional dimensions of each telehealth nurse's specific role. These behaviors include activities related to:
- Ethics
- Professional Development
- Research and Evidence-Based Practice
- Performance Improvement
- Communication
- Leadership
- Collaboration
- Professional Practice Evaluation
- Resource Utilization
- Environment

STANDARD 1

Assessment

▶ Standard

The RN practicing telehealth nursing is solely responsible for the systematic collection and interpretation of data relating to the health needs and concerns of a patient, family, and/or caregiver.

▶ Competencies

Telehealth RNs:

1. Function independently in a highly collaborative environment, maintaining personal professional responsibility for assessing all symptom-based encounters.

2. Establish a therapeutic rapport by "connecting with" and "getting to know" the patient, family, and/or caregiver, and interacting with the patient directly whenever possible.

3. Determine patient's perception of his/her immediate needs and concerns, identifying the patient's desired course of action.

4. Identify and address, whenever possible, social determinants that might pose barriers to the provision of optimal care (e.g., language, culture, financial considerations, disabilities, and behavioral health issues).

5. Provide support and collaboration to patients, family, and caregivers as key strategies of telehealth nursing assessment.

6. Collect subjective and objective data from the patient, family, and/or caregiver, and other sources as available and necessary, utilizing critical thinking and interpreting data as collected.

7. Arrange data collected in a sequential manner to address anticipated or immediate needs of patients using critical nursing judgment.

8. Utilize critical thinking and clinical judgment to select and apply the appropriate decision support tools to each patient encounter.

9. Apply evidence-based decision support tools, instruments, and other resources relevant to the provision of nursing care utilizing telehealth technology, critical thinking, and clinical judgment.

10. Recognize that nursing judgment supersedes decision support tools.

11. Prioritize data collection activities based on the patient's condition, situation, preferences, relevant contextual factors, and identified health needs.

12. Analyze and synthesize available data, information, and nursing knowledge relevant to the presenting health situation to identify patterns and variances in health as well as gaps in care.

13. Utilize clinical reasoning when investigating, focusing, verifying, clarifying, comparing, ruling-out, and processing patient data and information.

14. Use critical thinking and clinical reasoning to interpret data collected during triage encounters.

15. Avoid accepting patient self-diagnosis during triage encounters.

16. Speak directly with the patient to improve accuracy and ensure direct assessment whenever possible.

17. Conduct adequate re-assessment of patient and situation with frequent and repeat triage encounter.

18. Document the information and data collected in a retrievable, understandable, and readable format.

Assessment

▶ **Additional Competencies for Nurse Executives, Administrators, and Managers**

Telehealth Nurse Executives, Administrators, and Managers:

1. Use evidence-based practice guidelines and decision support tools to determine and/or refine data collection and analytic processes.
2. Identify essential elements of assessment and documentation for practice setting.
3. Evaluate assessment practices to ensure timely, reliable, valid, and adequate data collection and analysis.
4. Establish training, education, and resources on evidence-based assessment techniques for all nursing staff providing care utilizing telehealth technology.
5. Ensure information systems are in place that support the input and retrieval of reliable patient data.
6. Establish assessment expectations and monitor individual nursing staff performance.

Nursing Diagnoses

▶ Standard

Telehealth RNs analyze the assessment data to determine the nursing diagnostic statements for health promotion, health maintenance, or health-related problems or issues.

▶ Competencies

Telehealth RNs:

1. Identify the nursing diagnoses, actual or potential, based on the analysis of assessment data and information, current telehealth nursing knowledge, and evidence-based practice(s).
2. State the nursing diagnoses using standardized language, and understandable and recognized terminology utilizing clinical decision support tools.
3. Determine the nature and urgency of patient's symptom-based problem, without prejudgment and in accord with interpretation of subjective and objective data obtained during the nursing triage assessment.
4. Validate nursing diagnoses and/or issues with the patient, caregivers, and other members of the interprofessional health care team when appropriate.
5. Prioritize the nursing diagnoses based on the patient's condition, expectations and preferences, situation, cultural and age-specific considerations, and/or anticipated needs.
6. Documents clearly the nursing diagnoses to facilitate determination of expected outcomes and plan.
7. Identify actual or potential risks to the patient's health and safety or barriers to health, which may include but are not limited to interpersonal, systematic, or environmental circumstances.

▶ Additional Competencies for Nurse Executives, Administrators, and Managers

Telehealth Nurse Executives, Administrators, and Managers:

1. Provide educational opportunities and resources for professional nurses to develop competency and skill in the utilization of nursing diagnostic statements related to telehealth.
2. Promote an organizational climate that supports the validation of nursing diagnostic statements relevant to telehealth nursing.
3. Facilitate data analysis and decision-making processes to define practice patterns.

Outcomes Identification

▶ Standard

Telehealth RNs identify desired outcomes in an individualized plan of care specific to the patient, group, or population.

▶ Competencies

Telehealth RNs:

1. Derive desired outcomes and care dispositions from assessment and diagnosis(es).
2. Involve patient, family, and/or caregiver, and other health care providers in making shared decisions about formulating desired outcomes.
3. Consider associated risks, benefits, costs, current scientific evidence, and clinical expertise when formulating desired outcomes.
4. Define desired outcomes in terms of the patient's values; preferences; spiritual, cultural, and ethical considerations; age-related implications; situational environment; current scientific evidence; and telehealth best practices.
5. Develop desired outcomes that provide direction for continuity of care.
6. Modify desired outcomes based on changes in the status of patient or situation.

▶ Additional Competencies for Nurse Executives, Administrators, and Managers

Telehealth Nurse Executives, Administrators, and Managers:

1. Participate in the design and development of interprofessional processes that establish and maintain standards consistent with desired outcomes.
2. Support identification, development, and utilization of databases that include nurse-sensitive indicators, metrics, and quality outcomes.

Planning

▶ Standard

The RN practicing in a telehealth setting develops a plan that identifies strategies and alternatives to attain expected outcomes in individuals and/or populations.

▶ Competencies

Telehealth RNs:

1. Collaboratively develop an individualized plan of care for patients seeking care for health promotion, health maintenance, or health-related situational problems.
2. Apply current nursing knowledge and evidence-based nursing practice in the development of the plan of care.
3. Use professional nursing judgment to supersede triage decision support tool recommendation when clinically indicated.
4. Err on the side of caution if in doubt when determining disposition during triage encounters.
5. Include the patient, family, and/or caregiver or caregivers as appropriate and the health care team in making shared decisions about plans of care.
6. Consider patient, groups, and/or population needs in terms of age, gender, race, cultural values and practices, ethical and legal considerations, environmental factors, social determinants of health, and anticipated risks and benefits of interventions for individualized plan of care development.
7. Develop a timeline for plan of care implementation and goal achievement, reevaluation or reassessment, follow-up care, and care coordination as appropriate.
8. Ensure plan of care recommendations reflect current rules, regulations, and statutes.
9. Consider the most cost-effective, economic impact of the plan of care on patient and family resources.
10. Document plan of care and patient's progress to ensure continuity of care using recognized terminology.
11. Provide a plan of care that is understandable and acceptable to patient, family, and/or caregiver.
12. Validate plan of care is understood by patient, family, and/or caregiver.

▶ Additional Competencies for Nurse Executives, Administrators, and Managers

Telehealth Nurse Executives, Administrators, and Managers:

1. Facilitate development and improvement of organizational systems in which plans of care related to telehealth nursing practice are developed, documented, and evaluated.
2. Facilitate development and continuous improvement of mechanisms for plans of care to be recorded, reviewed, evaluated, and updated.
3. Ensure integration of organizational and management practices, nursing knowledge, standards, and guidelines into the telehealth plan of care process.
4. Support staff in developing and maintaining competency in the telehealth planning process.
5. Support telehealth nurses in deviating from the recommended triage decision support tool disposition when clinically indicated by patient's individual circumstances.
6. Collaborate with appropriate departments and/or disciplines so the organizational system operates effectively and efficiently to achieve improved outcomes.
7. Assure telehealth policies and procedures reflect current organizational, state, and federal rules, regulations, and statutes.

Implementation

▶ Standard

The RN practicing in the telehealth setting identifies with the patient how to implement the plan of care.

▶ Competencies

Telehealth RNs:

1. Prioritize interventions based on patient's health status, preferences, resources, motivation, and anticipated needs.
2. Facilitate implementation of plan of care in partnership with patient, caregivers, and health care team in a safe, efficient, and timely manner.
3. Implement unique telehealth knowledge, skills, attitudes, and competencies to develop interventions that promote wellness, restore health, and support end-of-life care.
4. Apply evidence-based, telehealth-specific interventions to achieve agreed upon outcomes during virtual encounters according to state regulations, regulatory agency standards, and appropriate organizational policies and procedures.
5. Provide interventions that are age appropriate, population specific, compassionate, holistic, and culturally sensitive with a focus on patient's communication and learning preferences.
6. Facilitate continuity of care in all nurse-patient telehealth encounters.
7. Utilize available technology to implement plan of care.
8. Document telehealth interventions and services provided in the patient record, including modifications, changes, or omissions of identified plan (ANA, 2015a).
9. Advocate for the health needs of individuals and diverse populations across the lifespan and continuum of care.

▶ Additional Competencies for Nurse Executives, Administrators, and Managers

Telehealth Nurse Executives, Administrators, and Managers:

1. Establish and promote organizational processes, systems, and resources to effectively implement plans of care.
2. Lead and facilitate change in organizations to improve implementation of evidence-based telehealth nursing interventions and strategies.
3. Lead and collaborate in improvement and adoption of information systems that facilitate accurate and complete documentation of telehealth nursing care.
4. Integrate quality improvement principles in organizational standards and policies that affect implementation of nursing plans of care.
5. Serve as an expert resource and consultant in assuring standards of telehealth nursing practice are integrated into organizations and health systems.
6. Collaborate with appropriate departments and other professionals in developing integrated systems that support ambulatory nursing care delivery.

Care Coordination/Transition Management

▶ Standard

The telehealth RN in the care coordination and transition management (CCTM) role coordinates delivery of care within the practice setting and across health care settings.

▶ Competencies

Telehealth RNs:

1. Demonstrate accountability across the virtual environment in maintaining continuity of care.
2. Facilitate patients' and/or populations' progress toward positive clinical outcomes.
3. Utilize an interprofessional approach to engage patients, caregivers, and providers in implementing the plan of care across care settings.
4. Facilitate transition of patients/populations to appropriate level of care.
5. Educate and activate patients and caregivers for optimal disease management by promoting healthy lifestyle changes and risk-reduction strategies in the prevention of illness across population(s).
6. Recognize and maximize virtual opportunities to increase quality of care.
7. Coordinate care for high-risk individuals and/or population(s) with the aim of preventing or delaying adverse outcomes.
8. Communicate relevant information across the care continuum to patients, caregivers, and interprofessional health care team.
9. Apply effective teamwork and collaboration skills to produce quality and effective patient outcomes.

▶ Additional Competencies for Nurse Executive, Administrators, and Managers

Telehealth Nurse Executive, Administrators, and Managers:

1. Plan global CCTM functions that meet the population's needs and are sustainable for the health care system.
2. Establish CCTM practice standards for evidence-based telehealth care delivery.
3. Communicate and build relationships with applicable stakeholders across the care continuum.
4. Develop and validate telehealth staff competencies consistent with CCTM standards of nursing practice and organizational policies.
5. Ensure compliance with external regulatory and accrediting organization(s).

Health Teaching and Health Promotion

▶ Standard

The RN practicing in the telehealth setting employs educational strategies that promote individual, community, and population health and safety.

▶ Competencies

Telehealth RNs:

1. Orient patient, family, and/or caregiver to the health care delivery system, services, access to care, and available resources.

2. Support patient and caregivers in developing skills for self-efficacy to promote, maintain, or restore health, such as healthy lifestyle tips, risk-reduction behaviors, age and developmental needs, daily living activities, and preventive care.

3. Utilize health teaching and health-promotion strategies that support the patient's learning needs, values, preferred language, socioeconomic status, and cultural and spiritual preferences.

4. Assess learning needs, abilities, readiness, preferences, and barriers to learning.

5. Incorporate patient's and/or caregiver's ability to understand and participate in the plan of care.

6. Use shared decision-making strategies to set goals. Goals should be specific, measurable, attainable, realistic, and timely.

7. Support patient and caregivers in developing skills for self-efficacy to promote, maintain, or restore health, such as healthy lifestyle and risk-reducing behavior.

8. Ensure patient, family, and/or caregiver understand risks and benefits and have an emergency plan in place.

9. Accurately document assessments, education, and interventions as well as modifications to the patient's plan of care to include patient understanding and agreement.

10. Provide accurate and timely information to support patient and caregivers in navigating the health care delivery system, including services, access to care, and available resources.

11. Maximize available technology to provide health-promotion disease-prevention strategies in both acute and chronic care management for optimal patient outcomes.

12. Remain knowledgeable regarding current population health recommendations to provide accurate, evidence-based anticipatory guidance to patients.

13. Promote and practice healthy self-care activities and stress management strategies and advocate for organizational policies and programs that promote a healthy workplace environment.

Health Teaching and Health Promotion

▶ **Additional Competencies for Nurse Executive, Administrators, and Managers**

Telehealth Nurse Executive, Administrators, and Managers:

1. Serve as role models for healthy self-care activities and stress management.
2. Create environments that promote positive, collegial staff and patient-staff interactions.
3. Provide guidelines and direction assuring consistency in care and operations.
4. Engage in a systematic evaluation of nursing educational processes and practices on a regular and on-going basis.
5. Utilize current evidence-based frameworks to design and implement health education information and programs.
6. Collaborate with interprofessional teams to promote health education.
7. Assure nursing staff receives appropriate and up-to-date training to help maximize their teaching, coaching, and motivational interviewing skill set.
8. Utilize data analysis for tracking and reporting clinical outcomes.

Consultation

▶ Standard

Telehealth RNs provide consultation in developing interprofessional plans of care, enhancing the ability of other professionals, and effecting change.

▶ Competencies

Telehealth RNs:

1. Synthesize clinical data, theoretical frameworks, evidence-based and best practices when providing consultation across the care continuum, while on the telephone, or through use of other telehealth technologies.
2. Communicate consult recommendations with appropriate stakeholders.

▶ Additional Competencies for Nurse Executive, Administrators, and Managers

Telehealth Nurse Executive, Administrators, and Managers:

1. Facilitate effectiveness of a consultation by involving the telehealth RN, members of the interprofessional team, and other stakeholders to enhance the decision-making process and assignment of role responsibilities.

Evaluation

▶ Standard

The RN practicing in the telehealth setting evaluates progress toward attainment of stated outcomes.

▶ Competencies

Telehealth RNs:

1. Conduct systematic, ongoing, and criteria-based evaluation of patient and/or population outcomes prescribed by plan of care and indicated timeline.
2. Integrate current evidence-based care into the telehealth evaluation process.
3. Include patient, family, and/or caregiver and members of interprofessional care team involved in the evaluation process.
4. Consider patient and family values, preferences, political, religious, cultural, environmental, and socioeconomic factors in evaluating the expected plan of care outcomes.
5. Reevaluate and revise the expected outcomes and plan of care as indicated.
6. Document patient status, evidence of patient, family, and/or caregiver participation and responses, including rationale for revision of plan of care.
7. Disseminate results of the nurse's evaluation to the patient, family, and/or caregiver, and others involved in the care or situation in accordance with state and federal laws, regulations, and organizational policies

▶ Additional Competencies for Nurse Executives, Administrators, and Managers

Telehealth Nurse Executives, Administrators, and Managers:

1. Facilitate the collaboration between telehealth nurses and interprofessional care team members to enhance the evaluation process through development of analytical tools.
2. Synthesize the evaluation results and their effect on telehealth nursing practice and patient and/or population outcomes.
3. Use research findings, evidence-based guidelines, standards, and evaluation results to improve care, services, and outcomes.
4. Advocate and encourage telehealth RNs in decision making related to evaluation process.
5. Communicate outcomes with other telehealth professionals through publications and presentations.

STANDARD 7

Ethics

▶ **Standard**

The RN practicing in the telehealth environment incorporates professional codes of ethics with compassion and respect for the inherent dignity, worth, and unique attributes of every person.

▶ **Competencies**

Telehealth RNs:

1. Apply knowledge of principles contained in ANA's (2015b) *Code of Ethics for Nurses with Interpretive Statements* as evidenced by nursing care and professional interactions.

2. Engage in activities that promote an ethical environment for provision of patient care and interactions with co-workers.

3. Participate in the identification and resolution of ethical concerns incorporating nursing's professional code of ethics and organizational policies.

4. Actively engage in addressing ethical concerns of patients, colleagues, or systems through dialogue with nursing colleagues, nursing managers, and involving organizational ethics entities when appropriate.

5. Maintain awareness of emerging ethical trends that affect patient rights in a telehealth setting.

6. Demonstrate activities consistent with self-efficacy through personal and professional growth.

7. Deliver nursing care that reflects the cultural, spiritual, intellectual, educational, and psychosocial differences of individual patients, families, or communities, and that preserves patient autonomy, dignity, and rights.

8. Provide information to facilitate informed decision making by the patient, family, and/or caregiver.

9. Ensure patients have opportunities to voice opinions, without fear of recrimination, regarding care and services received, and to have these issues reviewed and resolved per organizational policy and regulatory guidelines.

10. Incorporate appropriate measures to deliver safe patient care in cases where patients are not able to act in their own best interest or may not understand the potential consequences of their decisions.

11. Educate and support patients' self-efficacy skills.

12. Serve as the patient's advocate preserving the Patient Bill of Rights.

13. Demonstrate therapeutic interactions with patents and effective interactions with colleagues/staff while maintaining professional boundaries.

14. Disclose any observed illegal or incompetent practices including decisions made by impaired or potentially impaired personnel to supervisory leadership, appropriate professional bodies, and reporting agencies.

▶ **Additional Competencies for Nurse Executives, Administrators, and Managers**

Telehealth Nurse Executives, Administrators, and Managers:

1. Model ethical practices in all business and patient care interactions, including adherence to regulatory and professional ethical and practice standards.

2. Delineate in written policies patient rights and responsibilities related to confidentiality of information, personal privacy, and self-determination.

3. Create and implement policies that reflect the inherent self-worth, respect, and rights that everyone has to quality health care.

4. Create environments that support the discussion of decisions that address ethical risks, benefits, and outcomes for patients and staff.

Professional Development

▶ Standard

The RN practicing in the telehealth setting continually attains and updates knowledge and competency that reflects current telehealth nursing practice.

▶ Competencies

Telehealth RNs:

1. Pursue education and professional experiences that expand telehealth nursing knowledge, skills, and competencies.
2. Participate in ongoing, diverse educational activities related to appropriate telehealth nursing and health care knowledge, health system effectiveness, informatics, and professional issues.
3. Use current research findings and other evidence to expand professional and telehealth nursing knowledge.
4. Demonstrate a commitment to lifelong learning through self-reflection and inquiry to identify learning needs.
5. Seek experiences and acquire knowledge that reflect current practice to maintain skills and competence in telehealth nursing, clinical, and professional practice.
6. Actively seek, encourage, and support certification in a clinical specialty.
7. Maintain personal professional records that include evidence of current licensure, evaluation, and validation of clinical competence, continuing education, and certification.
8. Promote strength and effectiveness of the telehealth nursing profession through membership and active participation in professional and community organizations.
9. Mentor, support, and recruit new nurses to the telehealth nursing setting, incorporating them into professional development activities and ongoing continuing education.

▶ Additional Competencies for Nurse Executives, Administrators, and Managers

Telehealth Nurse Executives, Administrators, and Managers:

1. Ensure educational and professional development opportunities are available for continued nursing knowledge development, competency validation, and evidence-based nursing practice.
2. Ensure employee records provide evidence of competency and lifelong learning.
3. Encourage, reward, and recognize nurse certification in a specialty area.
4. Advocate for and support attainment of advanced degrees in nursing.
5. Promote organizational policies that support nursing education opportunities.
6. Mentor telehealth nurses to participate in educational conferences and active membership within professional organizations.
7. Partner with schools of nursing to provide an environment for students that is conducive to actively learning principles and practices of telehealth in ambulatory care nursing.
8. Ensure access to evidence-based journals and other clinical resources.
9. Ensure RNs new to telehealth nursing practice receive a comprehensive evidence-based orientation or residency program.

Research and Evidence-Based Practice

▶ Standard

The RN practicing in the telehealth setting actively participates in evidence-based practice initiatives and research activities to advance telehealth nursing and improve patient outcomes.

▶ Competencies

Telehealth RNs:

1. Review and evaluate current research and other literature for evidence relevant to telehealth nursing practice.
2. Utilize current research findings and other evidence to expand professional knowledge, enhance role performance, and increase understanding of telehealth nursing professional issues.
3. Identify clinical problems related to patient care delivery and/or telehealth nursing practice.
4. Evaluate the research evidence using criteria for scientific merit and optimal application in telehealth nursing practice settings.
5. Disseminate relevant telehealth evidence and research findings across organizational, community, and professional forums.
6. Integrate telehealth evidence and research findings into clinical practice.
7. Perform ongoing evaluation of the outcomes of evidence-based telehealth interventions.
8. Initiate, support, and/or participate in research studies of telehealth nursing practice.

▶ Additional Competencies for Nurse Executives, Administrators, and Managers

Telehealth Nurse Executives, Administrators, and Managers:

1. Institute strategies that facilitate the utilization of research as a basis for professional telehealth nursing practice.
2. Use evidence-based and best practices in the development of policies, procedures, and guidelines for telehealth nursing practice.
3. Ensure research conducted in the clinical and/or organizational environment undergoes review and approval by an institutional review board and adheres to ethical principles.
4. Validate research studies align with organizational and national health care priorities for applicability to telehealth nursing practice.
5. Advocate and facilitate nursing staff participation in learning opportunities, organizational quality and performance improvement activities, and relevant research initiatives that advance the delivery of telehealth nursing across the health care continuum.
6. Promote the integration of research findings into telehealth nursing practice.
7. Balance costs and benefits to patients, staff, and the organization of participation in research studies.
8. Advocate for organizational resources that enable nurses to learn and participate in nursing research and scholarly inquiry.
9. Actively participate in studies that offer potential for enhancing patient care delivery and care outcomes, telehealth nursing practice, and organizational/system effectiveness.
10. Support and encourage nurse researchers to disseminate findings utilizing activities such as presentations, publications, and consultations as well as through professional nursing organizations and educational opportunities.
11. Reward and recognize staff for participating in evidence-based practice and research activities.

Performance Improvement

▶ Standard

The RN practicing telehealth nursing enhances the quality, efficiency, and effectiveness of clinical and professional nursing practice within his/her clinical setting and organization.

▶ Competencies

Telehealth RNs:

1. Continuously evaluate telehealth nursing practice to identify opportunities for improving clinical outcomes, safety, and patient experience.
2. Participate in the identification and definition of nurse-sensitive indicators.
3. Lead and/or participate in quality and performance improvement initiatives within the organization and across the care continuum.
4. Evaluate and disseminate the findings of quality and performance improvement initiatives.
5. Implement evidence-based improvements into telehealth clinical, organizational, and professional practice.
6. Foster an environment that encourages patients, families, caregivers, visitors, and staff to provide input for patient care improvement activities.
7. Create and maintain a just culture through transparent communication, nondiscriminatory and equitable human resource practices, as well as judicious use of human and material resources.
8. Mitigate actual or potential risks to patient and staff safety.

▶ Additional Competencies for Nurse Executives, Administrators, and Managers

Telehealth Nurse Executives, Administrators, and Managers:

1. Solicit input from staff, patients, and families to identify strategies that improve patient care and organizational services.
2. Lead the development, implementation, and evaluation of current and innovative care delivery models.
3. Identify opportunities and establish priorities to continuously improve nursing quality of care and organizational performance.
4. Establish and communicate expectations for staff to participate in performance improvement initiatives.
5. Provide resources and opportunities to implement quality of care and performance improvement activities.
6. Foster interprofessional communication, collaboration, and coordination of improvement efforts.
7. Mentor, recognize, and reward nurses who participate in quality improvement activities.
8. Ensure systematic aggregation and analysis of quality data and use of appropriate statistical tools and techniques.
9. Trend and benchmark data to identify variances and improve the quality, efficiency, and effectiveness of care, and patient safety and satisfaction.
10. Mitigate actual and potential risks to patients and staff safety at the leadership level.
11. Advocate for integration of quality improvement activities that foster excellence in nursing care into the organizational strategic plan.
12. Evaluate efficiency and effectiveness of quality nursing care across the care continuum.
13. Partner with colleagues to conduct joint quality improvement initiatives.

Performance Improvement

▶ Additional Competencies for Nurse Executives, Administrators, and Managers

Telehealth Nurse Executives, Administrators, and Managers:

14. Advocate for the identification and adoption of nurse-sensitive indicators and metrics that identify the value of nursing in improved patient/population care and outcomes.

15. Create an environment that recognizes and rewards nursing excellence.

16. Facilitate professional nurse participation in monitoring and evaluating nursing care in accordance with established professional, regulatory, and organizational standards of practice.

17. Establish and continuously improve clinical guidelines that provide continuity of care within available resources.

Communication

▶ Standard

The RN practicing in the telehealth setting communicates effectively using a variety of formats, tools, and technologies to build professional relationships and to deliver care across the continuum.

▶ Competencies

Telehealth RNs:

1. Promote active communication using techniques that enhance learning and sharing of information.
2. Identify and evaluate personal skills and styles of communication to enhance effectiveness.
3. Share telehealth nursing best practices with peers, requesting feedback and evaluation.
4. Maintain professional communications and collaboration with all members of the interprofessional health care team and other stakeholders to improve coordination of care.
5. Contribute to a positive environment that fosters information sharing and learning.
6. Seek opportunities to create mentoring relationships among telehealth RNs.
7. Communicate knowledge and skills acquired through formal and informal professional development activities.
8. Exemplify a positive attitude and professional nursing practice that fosters a sense of excellence and enthusiasm among peers and colleagues.
9. Encourage trust with the patient, family, and/or caregiver by adhering to all privacy regulations.
10. Ensure information is communicated in a culturally sensitive manner.

▶ Additional Competencies for Nurse Executives, Administrators, and Managers

Telehealth Nurse Executives, Administrators, and Managers:

1. Foster a positive environment of collegiality and trust through shared interprofessional communication, experience, and decision making.
2. Seek, evaluate, and implement communication tools and technologies that improve telehealth nursing interactions and promote positive outcomes.
3. Act as a resource and role model for positive, professional communication with all members of the interprofessional care team across the health care continuum.
4. Recognize individual accomplishments and skills of telehealth RNs to foster a sense of professional pride, departmental expertise, and information sharing.
5. Influence professional and organization decision making to formulate standards that enhance telehealth nursing practice, environment, and outcomes.
6. Communicate intra- and interprofessionally that telehealth nursing is a unique domain of specialty nursing practice.

Leadership

▶ Standard

The RN practicing in the telehealth setting demonstrates leadership behaviors in practice settings, across the profession, and in the community.

▶ Competencies

Telehealth RNs:

1. Demonstrate respect for the dignity, worth, and contributions of others.
2. Assume an active leading role as a team player and team builder to create and maintain healthy, safe work environments in practice and community settings.
3. Recognize, address, and mitigate workflow inefficiencies.
4. Proactively anticipate and recognize the needs of others, using positive interactions and creative solutions to achieve effective outcomes.
5. Actively advocate for collegial, safe environments in telehealth clinical practice, organizational environments, and community settings.
6. Mentor newly assigned telehealth personnel and students contributing to a positive environment that fosters an attitude of information sharing and learning.
7. Assume responsibility and accountability for coordinating all aspects of the nursing process including delegated tasks consistent with their defined roles, nursing practice regulations, and professional standards.
8. Lead and participate in process improvement teams, committees, and activities related to telehealth practice in clinical, organizational, and community settings.
9. Collaborate with the interprofessional health care team to build and maintain effective and dynamic professional relationships.
10. Utilize critical-thinking skills to understand, address, and learn from experiences by self and others, thereby establishing an environment of trust, collaboration, and continuous learning.
11. Participate actively in organizational shared decision making that improves telehealth nursing practice, organizational performance, and outcomes.
12. Promote the continued personal advancement and effectiveness of professional telehealth nursing through membership and active participation in professional and community organizations.
13. Cultivate a culture of safety by sharing interactions related to errors, hazards, or problems that have the potential to negatively affect patients, families, and/or caregivers.
14. Collaborate with colleague by sharing knowledge and skills obtained through attendance at professional conferences, telehealth seminars, and membership in professional telehealth nursing organizations.

▶ Additional Competencies for Nurse Executives, Administrators, and Managers

Telehealth Nurse Executives, Administrators, and Managers:

1. Inspire nursing staff with a shared vision and direction for continuous quality improvement.
2. Lead and support activities that improve telehealth nursing practice, organizational performance, and healthy patient outcomes.
3. Build learning environments addressing shared decision making, evidence-based practice, organizational strategic direction, and advances in the health care industry.
4. Lead small and large-scale evidence-based change that is sensitive to organizational culture and values and perspectives of personnel.

Leadership

▶ Additional Competencies for Nurse Executives, Administrators, and Managers

Telehealth Nurse Executives, Administrators, and Managers:

5. Utilize transformational leadership to inspire shared practice and professional accountability.

6. Utilize conflict management skills to mediate professional and telehealth workplace issues resulting in mutually acceptable resolutions.

7. Acknowledge and reward contributions of telehealth RNs and high-performing teams.

8. Influence decision-making bodies to formulate standards that enhance telehealth nursing and health care practices, expand health system capabilities, and improve the health of individuals and the community.

9. Create a culture of safety that fosters reporting of unsafe conditions without fear of reprisal.

10. Advocate for and promulgate widespread use of quality measures and health information technologies that facilitate telehealth nursing practice efficiency, achievement of quality outcomes, and improved patient and population management.

11. Lead strategic, operational, and financial plans that impact delivery of telehealth nursing services.

12. Represent telehealth nursing on appropriate decision-making boards and committees of the organization to provide input on program planning and system changes that impact telehealth nursing care delivery and patient care outcomes.

13. Contribute to the expansion of telehealth nursing practice through membership and leadership in professional nursing organizations (Chassin & Loeb, 2011).

Collaboration

▶ Standard

The RN practicing in the telehealth setting collaborates with patients, family members, caregivers, and other health professionals in the conduct of nursing practice.

▶ Competencies

Telehealth RNs:

1. Communicate openly with patient, family, and/or caregiver and other health care professionals regarding the telehealth RN role in the provision of care.

2. Collaborate with other professionals regarding the promotion, prevention, and restoration of health through appropriate assessment and management of health-related problems.

3. Partner with patient, family, and/or caregiver and other healthcare professionals to develop a documented plan of care that promotes positive patient outcomes.

4. Use effective professional communication skills and tools to acquire and disseminate relevant information to patient, family, and/or caregiver and interprofessional team across the care continuum.

5. Identify gaps in care and collaborate with colleagues for resolution to achieve positive patient outcomes.

6. Share knowledge and skills with peers and colleagues as evidenced by such activities as patient care conferences or presentations at formal or informal meetings.

7. Proactively recognize the needs of others using positive interactions and creative solutions to achieve effective outcomes.

8. Collaborate with peers using shared decision making to implement the scope of telehealth nursing practice(s) and standards.

▶ Additional Competencies for Nurse Executives, Administrators, and Managers

Telehealth Nurse Executives, Administrators, and Managers:

1. Collaborate with professional nursing staff, using shared decision making, to implement policies and procedures that support the scope of telehealth nursing practice and standards across the organization.

2. Collaborate with colleagues to formulate strategic, operational, and financial plans that:
   • Establish the parameters and allocate the resources required to deliver safe, evidence-based, affordable, culturally competent, and age-relevant telehealth nursing care.
   • Maintain communication conduits that promote nurse collaboration with other health care team members.

3. Cultivate relationships that ensure representation of nursing on organizational decision-making boards and committees.

4. Collaborate at all levels of the organization to create an environment of professional excellence, transparency, and continuous learning.

5. Encourage the telehealth RN to identify operational issues that impact use of clinical scope and standards, organizational policies, and decision-support tools.

6. Develop and maintain a mechanism to ensure community resource lists are available and updated.

Professional Practice Evaluation

▶ Standard

The RN practicing in telehealth roles and/or settings evaluates his/her own and others' nursing practice in relation to professional practice standards and guidelines, patient outcomes, organizational policies and procedures, and relevant governmental regulations and statutes.

▶ Competencies

Telehealth RNs:

1. Utilize ongoing and systematic evaluations of telehealth work processes and individual performance standards.
2. Take action to achieve goals identified during professional telehealth practice evaluation processes.
3. Use evidence-based rationale for telehealth practice decisions and actions as part of informal and formal professional practice evaluations.
4. Engage in evaluation of self and other professional telehealth nursing staff to improve telehealth nursing practice and the patient experience.
5. Engage in regular organizational performance reviews to identify strengths, opportunities for growth, and set performance goals and objectives for self and telehealth professional practice.
6. Use available organizational systems, policies, and tools to review and evaluate telehealth nursing practice.
7. Take responsibility for periodic review and maintenance of one's professional portfolio.
8. Use independent nursing judgment, appropriate self-regulation, and professional accountability to evaluate telehealth practices.
9. Actively seek feedback regarding one's own telehealth nursing practice from patients, families, and professional colleagues.
10. Participate in department and organizational peer review, mentoring, and coaching regarding telehealth professional practice and/or role performance.

▶ Additional Competencies for Nurse Executives, Administrators, and Managers

Telehealth Nurse Executives, Administrators, and Managers:

1. Establish a culture of excellence within the organization through thoughtful consistent review and evaluation of telehealth evidence-based practices and quality measures within departments, in individual professional nurse practice, and during clinical training.
2. Institute a comprehensive process of telehealth employee performance appraisal that may encompass management feedback, peer reviews, patient and/or family comments, and interprofessional responses.
3. Support and facilitate staff involvement in the identification of telehealth best practices and clinical and ethical risk and legal issues.
4. Ensure staff involvement in the development of systematic approaches to evaluate and improve professional telehealth nursing practice.

Resource Utilization

▶ Standard

The RN practicing in the telehealth setting utilizes appropriate resources to plan, provide, and sustain evidence-based nursing services that are safe, effective, and fiscally responsible.

▶ Competencies

Telehealth RNs:

1. Partner with patients and caregivers to identify patient needs and resources available to achieve desired outcomes.
2. Delegate care-related activities to appropriate members of the care team following applicable laws and regulations when RN level of care is not required.
3. Advocate for the patient and caregiver(s) to access and implement appropriate and available resources to meet their health needs and concerns.
4. Evaluate the impact of resource allocation on the potential for harm, complexity of the task, and desired outcomes.
5. Educate and support the patient and caregiver(s) to become informed consumers about their options, costs, risks, and benefits of health care services.
6. Evaluate telehealth options related to safety, effectiveness, efficiency, and cost when two or more recommendations would result in the same expected patient outcome.

▶ Additional Competencies for Nurse Executives, Administrators, and Managers

Telehealth Nurse Executives, Administrators, and Managers:

1. Assess needs of population served and resources available to achieve desired health outcomes.
2. Design innovative solutions and ensure organizational resources are available to appropriately allocate and deploy telehealth technology based on evidence of effectiveness, efficiency, and potential for harm.
3. Ensure written organizational charts delineate nursing authority, accountability, chain of command, and lines of communication among nurses and other members of the interprofessional team.
4. Provide clearly defined, written position descriptions and performance standards for each category of nursing and assistive personnel that describes accountability for each employee's scope of practice and role within the interprofessional team.
5. Facilitate hiring and development of orientation plans for staff new to the telehealth role.
6. Implement a staffing plan advocating for the deployment of appropriate staff based on volume and complexity of care in accord with state nurse practice act and professional standards to deliver safe quality care that improves patient outcomes.
7. Create evaluation strategies that address cost effectiveness, cost benefits, and efficiency factors associated with nursing practice and staffing plan.

Environment

▶ Standard

The RN practicing in the telehealth setting actively engages in initiatives that create and maintain an environment of care that is safe and hazard-free.

▶ Competencies

Telehealth RNs:

1. Promote a safe and healthy workplace and professional practice environment.
2. Maintain professional practices and boundaries that ensure patients' privacy and protection of their health information through recognized standards of security and encryption.
3. Ensure patients are informed of their rights and responsibilities as it applies to a telehealth environment.
4. Assure telehealth equipment is used per manufacturer guidelines and meets environment of care standards.
5. Integrate into daily practice written policies and procedures that are specific to the environment of care.
6. Maintain access to and knowledge of emergency resources, contact numbers, and has contingency plan available.
7. In event of technology failure, back-up plan in place which outlines alternate method of communication between and among sites.

▶ Additional Competencies for Nurse Executives, Administrators, and Managers

Telehealth Nurse Executives, Administrators, and Managers:

1. Ensure an environment that is private and secure, and that maintains confidentiality of patient information and takes into consideration:
   a. Access and security of computer resources.
   b. Ergonomics and equipment (technologies).
   c. Lighting, space requirements, and environmental services.
   d. Sound transmission and issues of privacy and confidentiality.
   e. Accessibility of current references and resources.
   f. Security and personal safety with each telehealth interaction.
   g. Accessibility and functionality of an environment for staff with disabilities.
2. Assure written policies and procedures are available regarding confidentiality and care environment.
3. Implement policies and procedures that address personnel training, personal protective equipment, monitoring, reporting, the intervention process, and documentation of occurrences.
4. Assure written policies and procedures and ongoing monitoring are available regarding nurse's remote work environment.
5. Ensure home/remote work environment meets the same confidentiality, safety, security, and ergonomic expectations of an employer-provided work environment with documentation of monitoring frequency, findings, and actions.
6. Provide an ongoing safety program that includes education, monitoring, identification, prevention, and correction or safety and health hazards as appropriate to the work environment.

Environment

▶ **Additional Competencies for Nurse Executives, Administrators, and Managers**

Telehealth Nurse Executives, Administrators, and Managers:

7. Ensure staff attend and maintain documentation of compliance of required environment of care education and competencies.

8. Determine level of resources needed for safe, quality patient care that is compliant with applicable federal and state rules and regulations, organizational policies, and standards of telehealth nursing practice.

9. Provide an organizational chart that delineates nursing authority, accountability, and lines of communication among members of the health care team.

10. Provide written position descriptions that define responsibilities and performance measurements of telehealth nursing staff, congruent with applicable federal, state, territory, or commonwealth statutes, rules, regulations, and accepted standards of telehealth nursing practice.

11. Partner with other health care organizations and agencies to promote healthy communities.

Summary of Frequently Used Telehealth Terms

Term	Definition	Reference
Telehealth	The delivery, management, and coordination of health services that integrate electronic information and telecommunications technologies to provide access to health assessment, diagnosis, intervention, consultation, supervision, and information across distance.	Greenburg et al., 2003, p. 8
	Remote delivery of nursing care through technology for purposes of assessment, information exchange, clinical decision making, and providing nursing interventions.	Nagel, 2014, p. 392
	Telehealth is provided in several modalities, including but not limited to: • Real-time or synchronous communication such as telephone, webcam, or audio or video links. • The storage and forwarding of information, such as diagnostic imaging data. • Remote patient monitoring, such as at-home vital sign measurement of blood glucose level testing. • mHealth (mobile health), which can include the use of wearable devices, cell phones, or smartphone applications.	Brouse, 2016, p. 64
Virtual environment	An environment other than the one in which the participant is actually present, more usefully it is a computer-generated model where a participant can interact intuitively in real time with the environment or objects within it, and to some extent has a feeling of actually being there, or a feeling of presence.	Wilson, 1997, pp. 1057-1058
Telepresence	The sense of being physically present with virtual objects at the remote tele-operator site.	Sheridan, 1992, p. 120
Virtual presence	The sense of being physically present with visual, auditory, or force displays generated by a computer.	Sheridan, 1992, p. 120
Telehealth nursing	The delivery, management, and coordination or care and services provided via telecommunications technology within the domain of nursing.	Greenberg et al., 2003, pp. 8-9
	The telehealth nurse engages in the practice of nursing by interacting with a client at a remote site to electronically receive the client's health status, initiate and transmit therapeutic interventions and regimens, and monitor and record the client's response and nursing care outcomes. The value of telehealth to the client is increased access to skilled, empathetic, and effective nursing delivered through telecommunications technology.	NCBSN, 2014, p. 1
Telemedicine	The delivery, management, and coordination or care and services provided via telecommunications technology within the domain of medicine. Telemedicine is a broad term describing the subset of telehealth pertaining to the practice of medicine at a distance.	Greenberg et al., 2003, pp. 8-9
	Telemedicine, which may be used interchangeably with telehealth, is sometimes used to encompass a broader definition of health care that uses telecommunications technologies. Videoconferencing, transmission of still images and other data, e-health including patient portals, mHealth, remote monitoring, continuing medical education, and medical call centers are all considered part of telemedicine and telehealth.	American Telemedicine Association, 2014, p. 5
	Telemedicine meets the standards of traditional encounters: a clinician performs an evaluation, provides evidence-based recommendations, arranges follow-up, and documents the encounter in a medical record. Telemedicine also creates opportunities not present during traditional office encounters. Using video or web-based platforms, clinicians can see into a patient's home, assess the home environment risk factors, and talk to family members.	DeJong, Lucey, & Dudley, 2015, p. 2351

Glossary

Many terms in nursing and health care have multiple meanings and can be used in multiple contexts. Certain terms are defined to clarify the intent and application of these standards. Terms not defined are assumed either to have a generally acceptable meaning and interpretation, or to require contextual interpretation depending on the setting and application.

Adverse event – Unnecessary patient injury, harm, pain, suffering, or death resulting from either medical management or health system process rather than from illness or disease.

Advocacy – Act or process of advancing or supporting (a cause or proposal) on behalf of another.

Care continuum (continuum of care) – Over the course of the patient's life, the patient will receive health-related care from a variety of health care and service professionals in a variety of health care settings.

Care coordination – Deliberate organization of patient care activities between two or more participants (including the patient) involved in the patient's care to facilitate appropriate delivery of health care services. Organizing care involves the marshaling of personnel and other resources needed to carry out all required patient care activities and is often managed by exchange of information among participants responsible for different aspects of care.

Caregiver – Individual (e.g., family member, friend, or companion) over the age of 18 years who provides care and/or support.

Care transitions – Change in the level of service or location of providers of care as patients move within and across the health care system.

Clinical reasoning – Process by which nurses (and other clinicians) collect cues, process information, come to an understanding of a patient problem or situation, plan and implement interventions, evaluate outcomes, and reflect on and learn from the process (Levett-Jones et al., 2013).

Competency – Expected level of performance that integrates knowledge, skills, abilities, and judgment.

Collaboration – Working together toward a common goal; to pursue a common purpose and a sharing of knowledge and information to decide issues, resolve problems, and set goals within a structure and relationship of collegiality.

Competence – Ability to demonstrate knowledge, skills, and attitude as well as critical thinking and interpersonal skills necessary to perform one's role and job responsibilities.

Continuity of care – Health care that remains consistent or uninterrupted throughout the care process.

Critical thinking – Intellectually disciplined process of actively and skillfully conceptualizing, applying, analyzing, synthesizing, and/or evaluating information gathered from, or generated by, observation, experience, reflection, reasoning, or communication, as a guide to belief and action. This is demonstrated in nursing by exercising clinical judgment that also encompasses ethical, diagnostic, and therapeutic research dimensions (The Foundation for Critical Thinking, 2018).

Cultural competence – Requires developing cultural awareness (conscious learning process through which one becomes appreciative and sensitive to the cultures of other people), cultural knowledge (process of understanding key aspects of a group's culture), cultural skills (ability to collect relevant data for health histories and perform culturally specific assessments), and cultural encounters (process that encourages one to engage directly in cross-cultural interactions with people from culturally diverse backgrounds) (AAACN, 2013).

Decision support tools – A plan or guide for the assessment and management of a clinical problem to reduce the risk of omission and increase the predictability of desired clinical outcomes. The unique needs of patient preferences and his/her specific situation must be incorporated into their use in a practice setting. Protocols, guidelines, or algorithms may be referred to as decision support tools. Decision support tools are developed using scientifically valid and documented clinical principles and resources, clinical experience, and the needs of the setting in which they are used. They may be in hard copy or computerized format. They should be clinically reviewed annually and revised as needed (North et al., 2014).

Digital literacy – Ability to use information and communication technologies to find, evaluate, create, and communicate information, requiring both cognitive and technical skills (Visser, 2012).

Education process – Systematic planned course of action between and among professionals and patients to develop or expand health care knowledge and/or skills; it is a teaching-learning process among participants.

Electronic health record – Secure, real-time, point-of-care, patient-centric documentation system of patient care, services, and status that serves as an information resource for interprofessional clinicians.

Engagement in health care – Active and/or proactive behaviors that patients need to engage in to obtain the greatest benefit from available health care services.

Environment – Complex interrelationship of factors external to the organization and those within the health care organization that surround the patient/population and affects care delivery services.

Ergonomics – Scientific discipline concerned with the interactions between humans and other elements of a system, and the profession that applies theory, principles, data, and methods to system design in order to optimize human well-being and overall system performance (International Ergonomics Association, 2018).

Ethics – Philosophical framework for examining values as they relate to human behaviors: how behaviors are viewed as right or wrong, good or bad, and is concerned with both the motives and outcomes of actions and/or decisions.

Evidence-based practice – Conscientious, explicit, and judicious use of current best scientific evidence in making and implementing decisions addressing the care and services for patients and populations; nurses utilize research and clinical knowledge and expertise.

Expected outcomes – Anticipated results of health care treatments and/or services delivered to patients and/or populations seen as desirable, measurable, and observable behaviors.

Family – Family members are defined by the patient in her/his own terms and may include individuals related by blood, marriage, or in self-defined relationships. (This definition is intended to include the family in nursing care as appropriate. It is not intended as a legal definition of family.)

Hazardous conditions – Any set of circumstances (exclusive of the disease, disorder, or condition for which the patient is undergoing care, treatment, and services) defined by the organization that significantly increases likelihood of a serious adverse outcome.

Health care team – Includes patients, caregivers, and/or population members as well as providers within and across health care systems who partner in developing and implementing plans of care that improve health.

Health literacy – Degree to which individuals have the capacity to obtain, process, and understand basic health information and services needed to make appropriate health decisions (AAACN, 2017a, 2017b).

Infection control – System designed for surveillance, prevention, and control of infection.

Institutional review board (IRB) – Group of professionals convened by research institutions to ensure the protection of rights and welfare of human research subjects participating in research conducted under their auspices. IRBs make an independent determination to approve, require modifications in, or disapprove research protocols based on whether human subjects are adequately protected, as required by federal regulations and local institutional policy.

Interprofessional team – Group of individuals from different disciplines working and communicating with each other, providing his/her knowledge, skills, and attitudes to augment and support the contributions of others.

Lifelong learning – "The provision or use of both formal and informal learning opportunities throughout people's lives in order to foster the continuous development and improvement of the knowledge and skills needed for employment and personal fulfilment" (Collins English Dictionary, n.d.).

Literature reviews – Search and analysis of a body of research findings about a specific issue or topic.

Machine learning – Application of artificial intelligence that provides systems the ability to automatically learn and improve from experience without being explicitly programmed. Machine learning focuses on development of computer programs that can access data and use it learn for themselves (Rigla et al., 2017).

Nursing-sensitive indicators – Indicators that capture care or its outcomes most affected by nursing care (Heslop & Lu, 2014).

Outcomes – End results that are measurable, desirable, and observable and that transfer into observable behaviors (ANA, 2015a).

Patient – Person, client, family, group, community, or population who is the focus of attention and to whom the RN is providing services as sanctioned by the state regulatory bodies (ANA, 2015a).

Performance improvement – Systematic analysis of the structure, processes, and outcomes within health care systems for improving delivery of care and outcomes (AAACN, 2017a, 2017b).

Plan – Comprehensive outline of the components that need to be addressed to attain expected outcomes (ANA, 2015a).

Population health management – A means to organize systems of care for populations, identify and implement evidence-based interventions, and measure both short and long-term outcomes for both the individual and the population.

Quality of care – Degree to which ambulatory care nursing and health services for individuals, groups, and populations increase likelihood of achieving desired health outcomes and are consistent with current professional knowledge.

Quality control – Process that measures clinical and/or organizational performance and compares outcomes against goals and acts on the differences when performance falls short of defined goals.

Reflective practice – "Engaging in the process of reflecting on the development of knowledge and skills of a professional practice" (Bassot, 2016, p. 1).

Registered nurse (RN) – An individual nurse who is registered or licensed by a state, commonwealth, territory, government, or other regulatory body to practice as an RN (ANA, 2015a).

Research – Application of systematic, scientific methods to study phenomena and generate knowledge.

Safety – Degree to which the risk of an intervention and risk in the care environment are reduced for a patient and other person, including health care practitioners.

Self-efficacy – A person's confidence in his/her ability to carry out behaviors necessary to achieve the desired goal.

Social determinants of health – Conditions in the environment in which people are born, live, learn, work, play, worship, and age that affect a wide range of health, functioning, and quality-of-life outcomes and risks and may contribute to health inequities (WHO, 2017).

Standards – Authoritative statements defined and promoted by the profession by which quality of practice, service, or education can be evaluated (ANA, 2015a).

Standards of practice – Statements that describe a competent level of nursing care as demonstrated by the nursing process (ANA, 2015a).

Standards of professional performance – Statements that describe a competent level of behavior in the professional role (ANA, 2015a).

Telecommunications – Use of the telephone, Internet, interactive video, remote sensory devices, or robotics to transmit information from one site to another.

Telehealth – Delivery, management, and coordination of health services that integrate electronic information and telecommunications technologies to increase access, improve outcomes, and contain or reduce costs of health care. *Telehealth* is an umbrella term used to describe the wide range of services using technologies and delivered across distances by all health-related disciplines.

Telehealth nursing practice – Delivery, management, and coordination of care and services provided via telecommunications technology.

Telehealth nursing – Includes all care and services within the scope of nursing practice that are delivered over the telephone. It is a component of telehealth nursing practice restricted to the telephone. (Greenberg et al., 2003, pp. 8-9)

Telephone triage – An interactive process between nurse and client that occurs over the telephone and involves identifying the nature and urgency of client health care needs and determining the appropriate disposition. The telephone triage is an essential element of telehealth nursing that focuses on assessment, prioritization, and referral to the appropriate level of care (Greenberg, et al., 2003, pp. 8-9).

Unlicensed assistive personnel – Unlicensed individual who is trained to function in an assistive role to the licensed nurse in the provision of patient/client activities as delegated by the nurse.

Virtual environment – Environment other than the one in which the participant(s) is present (Nagel, 2014; Wilson, 1997).

Virtual health care – Electronically enabled care services, including clinician-to-clinician, provider-to patient, and consumer-driven interactions. This definition encompasses a range of terminologies including *telemedicine, telehealth, e-health,* and *mobile health* (Lefar, 2015).

Web-based sources of evidence – Multiple sites on the World Wide Web that contain research-based evidence.

Wellness – Integrated, congruent functioning aimed toward reaching one's highest potential (ANA, 2015a).

References

American Academy of Ambulatory Care Nursing (AAACN)/American Nurses Association (ANA). (1997). *Nursing in ambulatory care: The future is here.* Washington, DC: American Nurses Publishing.

American Academy of Ambulatory Care Nursing (AAACN). (2007). *Ambulatory care nursing administration and practice standards.* Pitman, NJ: Author.

American Academy of Ambulatory Care Nursing (AAACN). (2011). *Scope and standards of practice for professional telehealth nursing* (5th ed.). Pitman, NJ: Author.

American Academy of Ambulatory Care Nursing (AAACN). (2013). *Core curriculum for ambulatory care nursing* (3rd ed.). Pitman, NJ: Author.

American Academy of Ambulatory Care Nursing (AAACN). (2016). *Scope and standards of practice for RNs in care coordination and transition management.* Pitman, NJ: Author.

American Academy of Ambulatory Care Nursing (AAACN). (2017a). *Scope and standards of practice for professional ambulatory care nursing* (9th ed.). Pitman, NJ: Author.

American Academy of Ambulatory Care Nursing (AAACN). (2017b). Position statement on the role of the registered nurse in ambulatory care nursing. *Nursing Economic$, 35*(1), 39-47.

American Nurses Association (ANA). (2004). *Nursing scope and standards of practice* (2nd ed.). Silver Spring, MD: Author.

American Nurses Association (ANA). (2015a). *Nursing scope and standards of practice* (3rd ed.). Silver Spring, MD: Author.

American Nurses Association (ANA). (2015b). *Code of ethics for nurses with interpretive statements.* Silver Spring, MD: Author

American Nurses Association (ANA). (2012). *The essential guide to nursing practice: Applying ANA's scope and standards in practice and education.* Silver Spring, MD: Author.

American Recovery and Reinvestment Act of 2009, P.L. 111.5, 123 Stat. 115 (2009). Retrieved from https://www.gpo.gov/fdsys/pkg/PLAW-111publ5/pdf/PLAW-111publ5.pdf

American Telemedicine Association. (2014). *Standards - Maryland.* Retrieved from https://health.maryland.gov/mhqcc/Documents/Standards_Framework.pdf

Bassot, B. (2016). *The reflective practice guide: An interdisciplinary approach to critical reflection.* New York, NY: Routledge.

Brous, E. (2016). Legal considerations in telehealth and telemedicine. *American Journal of Nursing, 116*(9), 64-67.

Chassin, M.R., & Loeb, J.M. (2011). The ongoing quality improvement journey: Next stop, high reliability. *Health Affairs, 30*(4), 559-568.

Coleman, E.A., & Boult, C. (2003), Improving the quality of transitional care for persons with complex care needs. *Journal of the American Geriatrics Society, 51,* 556-557.

Collins English Dictionary. (n.d.). *Lifelong learning.* Retrieved from http://www.dictionary.com/browse/lifelong-learning

Darkins, A., & Carey, M. (2000). Telemedicine and telehealth: Principles, policies, performance, and pitfalls. *Choice Reviews Online, 38*(1).

Deblois, D., & Millefoglie, M. (2015). Telehealth. *Nursing Management, 46*(6), 10-12.

Dejong, C., Lucey, C.R., & Dudley, R.A. (2015). Incorporating a new technology while doing no harm, virtually. *JAMA, 314*(22), 2351.

Dinesen, B., Nonnecke, B., Lindeman, D., Toft, E., Kidholm, K., Jethwani, K., & Nesbitt, T. (2016). Personalized telehealth in the future: A global research agenda. *Journal of Medical Internet Research, 18*(3).

Flodgren, G., Rachas, A., Farmer, A.J., Inzitari, M., & Shepperd, S. (2015). Interactive telemedicine: Effects on professional practice and health care outcomes. *Cochrane Database of Systematic Reviews.* Retrieved from http://www.cochrane.org/CD002098/EPOC_interactive-telemedicine-effects-professional-practice-and-healthcare-outcomes

Greenberg, M.E., Espensen, M., Becker, C., & Cartwright, J. (2003). Telehealth nursing practice special interest group adopts teleterms. *AAACN Viewpoint, 25*(1), 8-10.

Guise, V., & Wiig, S. (2017). Perceptions of telecare training needs in home healthcare services: A focus group study. *BMC Health Services Research, 17*(1), 164.

Haas, S.A., Swan, B.A., & Haynes, T.S. (2014). *Care coordination and transition management core curriculum.* Pitman, NJ: American Academy of Ambulatory Care Nursing.

Heslop, L., & Lu, S. (2014). A concept analysis. *Journal of Advanced Nursing, 70*(11), 2469-2482.

Institute of Medicine (IOM). (2012). *The role of telehealth in an evolving health care environment: Workshop summary.* Washington, DC: National Academies Press.

International Ergonomics Association. (2018). *What is ergonomics?* Retrieved from http://www.iea.cc/whats/index.html

Lefar, S. (2015). *What's real in virtual health?* Retrieved from www.sg2.com/health-care-intelligence-blog/2015/03/whats-real-in-virtual-health/

Levett-Jones, T., Sundin, D., Bagnell, M., Hague, K., Schumann, W., Taylor, C., & Wink, J. (2013). *Learning to think like a nurse.* Retrieved from http://journals.sfu.ca/hneh/index.php/hneh/article/view/65

Lipstein, S.H., & Kellermann, A.L. (2016). Workforce for 21st-century health and health care. *JAMA, 316*(16), 1665.

Macy, J. (2016). RN: Partners in transforming primary care. *Macy Foundation Conference.* Atlanta, GA.

Mastel, M., Matlock, A.M., & Start, R. (2016). Ambulatory care nurse-sensitive indicators series: Capturing the role of nursing in ambulatory care – the case for meaningful nurse-sensitive indicators. *Nursing Economic$, 34*(2), 92-97, 76.

Nagel, D. (2014). Knowing the person in a virtual environment: Protocol for a grounded theory study of telehealth in nursing practice. *International Journal of Arts & Sciences, 7*(3), 377-394.

Nagel, D.A., & Penner, J. L. (2016). Conceptualizing telehealth in nursing practice. *Journal of Holistic Nursing, 34*(1), 91-104.

Nagel, D.A., Stacey, D., Momtahan, K., Gifford, W., Doucet, S., & Etowa, J. B. (2016). Getting a picture. *Journal of Holistic Nursing, 35*(1), 67-85.

National Council of State Boards of Nursing (NCSBN). (2017). *The nurse licensure compact. Unlocking access to nursing care across the nation.* Presentation at the Federal Trade Commission Workshop, Washington, DC. Retrieved from https://www.ftc.gov/system/files/documents/public_events/1224893/slides_-_katherine_thomas_ncsbn.pdf

National Council of State Boards of Nursing (NCSBN). (2014). *Position paper on telehealth nursing practice.* Retrieved from https://www.ncsbn.org/14_Telehealth.pdf

National Quality Forum. (2017). *Creating a framework to support measure development for telehealth.* Retrieved from https://www.qualityforum.org/Publications/2017/08/Creating_a_Framework_to_Support_Measure_Development_for_Telehealth.aspx

North, F., Richards, D.D., Bremseth, K.A., Lee, M.R., Cox, D.L., Varkey, P., & Stroebel, R.J. (2014). Clinical decision support improves quality of telephone triage documentation – an analysis of triage documentation before and after computerized clinical decision support. *BMC Medical Informatics & Decision Making, 14,* 20.

Omery, A. (2003). Advice nursing practice. *JONA: The Journal of Nursing Administration, 33*(6), 353-360.

Paschke, S.M., Witwer, S., Richards, W.C., Jessie, A., Harden, L., Martinez, K., & Vinson, M.H. (2017). The role of the registered nurse in ambulatory care. *Nursing Economic$, 35*(1), 39-47.

Patsalides, L. (2010). *A definition and teacher's contemplation of lifelong learners.* Retrieved from http:www.brighthub.com/hubfolio/laurie/-patsalides/articles/38286.aspx

Rigla, M., García-Sáez, G., Pons, B., & Hernando, M.E. (2017). Artificial intelligence methodologies and their application to diabetes. *Journal of Diabetes Science and Technology, 12*(2), 303-310. doi:10.1177/1932296817710475

Rutenberg, C., & Greenberg, M.E. (2012). *The art and science of telephone triage: How to practice nursing over the phone.* Hot Springs, AR: Telephone Triage Consulting, Inc.

Sharma, U., & Clarke, M. (2014). Nurses' and community support workers' experience of telehealth: A longitudinal case study. *BMC Health Services Research, 14,* 164.

Sheridan, T.B. (1992). Musings on telepresence and virtual presence. *Presence: Teleoperators and Virtual Environments, 1*(1), 120-126. doi:10.1162/pres.1992.1.1.120

The Foundation for Critical Thinking Community (2018). Retrieved from http://www.criticalthinking.org/pages/the-critical-thinking-community/744

The National Council of State Boards of Nursing (NCSBN®). (2014). *Position paper on telehealth nursing practice.* Retrieved from https://www.ncsbn.org/14_Telehealth.pdf

U.S. Department of Health and Human Services. (2018). *Healthy People 2020.* Retrieved from https://www.healthypeople.gov/

Vinson, M.H., McCallum, R., Thornlow, D.K., & Champagne, M.T. (2011). Design, implementation, and evaluation of population-specific telehealth nursing services. *Nursing Economic$, 29*(5), 265-272.

Visser, M. (2012). *Digital literacy definition.* Retrieved from http://connect.ala.org/node/181197

While, A., & Dewsbury, G. (2011). Nursing and information and communication technology (ICT): A discussion of trends and future directions. *International Journal of Nursing Studies, 48*(10), 1302-1310.

Wilson, J.R. (1997). Virtual environments and ergonomics: Needs and opportunities. *Ergonomics, 40*(10), 1057-1077.

World Health Organization (WHO). (2017) *Health impacts assessment.* Retrieved from http://www.who.int/hia/evidence/doh/en/

Additional Readings

Allen, M., Aylott, M., Loyola, M., Moric, M., & Saffarek, L. (2015). Nurses: Extending care through telehealth. *Studies in Health Technology and Informatics, 208,* 35-39.

Bartz, C., Hardiker, N.R., & Coenen, A. (2015). Toward a Global eHealth Observatory for Nursing. *Studies in Health Technology and Informatics, 216,* 1114.

Berkhof, F.F., Berg, J.W., Uil, S.M., & Kerstjens, H.A. (2014). Telemedicine, the effect of nurse-initiated telephone follow up, on health status and health-care utilization in COPD patients: A randomized trial. *Respirology, 20*(2), 279-285. doi:10.1111/resp.12437

Berman, S.J., Minatodani, D., & Jordan, P. J. (2012). Telehealth monitoring with nurse clinician oversight. *Archives of Internal Medicine, 172*(20), 1612. doi:10.1001/archinternmed.2012.4433

Black, J.T., Romano, P.S., Sadeghi, B., Auerbach, A.D., Ganiats, T.G., Greenfield, S., … Ong, M.K. (2014). A remote monitoring and telephone nurse coaching intervention to reduce readmissions among patients with heart failure: Study protocol for the Better Effectiveness After Transition - Heart Failure (BEAT-HF) randomized controlled trial. *Trials, 15*(1), 124. doi:10.1186/1745-6215-15-124

Bodenheimer, T., & Mason, D. (2016). *Registered nurses: Partners in transforming primary care.* Retrieved from http://macyfoundation.org/publications/publication/registered-nurses-partners-in-transforming-primary-care

Broderick, A. (2013). *The Veterans Health Administration: Taking home telehealth services to scale nationally.* Retrieved from http://www.commonwealthfund.org/publications/case-studies/2013/jan/telehealth-vha

Brunetti, N.D., Dellegrottaglie, G., Giuseppe, G.D., & Biase, M.D. (2014). Remote tele-medicine cardiologist support for care manager nursing of chronic cardiovascular disease: Preliminary report. *International Journal of Cardiology, 176*(2), 552-556. doi:10.1016/j.ijcard.2014.07.020

Cady, R.G., & Finkelstein, S. M. (2014). Task – Technology fit of video telehealth for nurses in an outpatient clinic setting. *Telemedicine and e-Health, 20*(7), 633-639. doi:10.1089/tmj.2013.0242

Carlson, J., Cohen, R., & Bice-Stephens, W. (2014, October-December). Effectiveness of telebehavioral health program nurse case managers. *U.S. Army Medical Department Journal,* 36-45.

Camargo, K.R. (2011). Closing the gap in a generation: Health equity through action on the social determinants of health. *Global Public Health, 6*(1), 102-105.

Coster, C.D., Quan, H., Elford, R., Li, B., Mazzei, L., & Zimmer, S. (2010). Follow-through after calling a nurse telephone advice line: A population-based study. *Family Practice, 27*(3), 271-278. doi:10.1093/fampra/cmq003

Côté, J., Rouleau, G., Ramirez-Garcia, P., & Bourbonnais, A. (2015). Virtual nursing intervention adjunctive to conventional care: The experience of persons living with HIV. *JMIR Research Protocols, 4*(4). doi:10.2196/resprot.4158

Craven, O., Hughes, C.A., Burton, A., Saunders, M.P., & Molassiotis, A. (2013). Is a nurse-led telephone intervention a viable alternative to nurse-led home care and standard care for patients receiving oral capecitabine? Results from a large prospective audit in patients with colorectal cancer. *European Journal of Cancer Care, 22*(3), 413-419. doi:10.1111/ecc.12047

Davis, K. (2014). Nurses' and community support workers' experience of telehealth: A longitudinal case study. *Primary Health Care, 24*(10), 18-18.

Demaerschalk, B.M., Kiernan, T.J., & Investigators, S. (2010). Vascular neurology nurse practitioner provision of telemedicine consultations. *International Journal of Telemedicine and Applications.* Retrieved from https://www.hindawi.com/journals/ijta/2010/507071/ doi:10.1155/2010/507071

Dinesen, B., Nonnecke, B., Lindeman, D., Toft, E., Kidholm, K., Jethwani, K., … Nesbitt, T. (2016). Personalized telehealth in the future: A global research agenda. *Journal of Medical Internet Research, 18*(3).

Duplaga, M. (2016). Searching for a role of nursing personnel in developing landscape of Ehealth: Factors determining attitudes toward key patient empowering applications. *Plos One, 11*(4). doi:10.1371/journal.pone.0153173

Dy, P., Morin, P.C., & Weinstock, R.S. (2013). Use of telemedicine to improve glycemic management in a skilled nursing facility: A pilot study. *Telemedicine and e-Health, 19*(8), 643-645. doi:10.1089/tmj.2012.0274

Espensen, M. (2009). *Telehealth nursing practice essentials.* Pitman, NJ: American Academy of Ambulatory Care Nursing.

Ferrara, A., Hedderson, M.M., Ching, J., Kim, C., Peng, T., & Crites, Y. M. (2012). Referral to telephonic nurse management improves outcomes in women with gestational diabetes. *Obstetrical & Gynecological Survey, 67*(10), 610-611. doi:10.1097/01.ogx.0000422942.56614.26

Frisch, N., Atherton, P., Borycki, E., Mickelson, G., Cordeiro, J., Lauscher, H.N., & Black, A. (2014). Growing a professional network to over 3000 members in less than 4 years: Evaluation of InspireNet, British Columbia's virtual nursing health services research network. *Journal of Medical Internet Research, 16*(2). doi:10.2196/jmir.3018

Gagnon, M., Paré, G., Pollender, H., Duplantie, J., Côté, J., Fortin, J., ... Malo, F. (2011). Supporting work practices through telehealth: Impact on nurses in peripheral regions. *BMC Health Services Research, 11*(1). doi:10.1186/1472-6963-11-27

Gray, L.C., Edirippulige, S., Smith, A.C., Beattie, E., Theodoros, D., Russell, T., & Martin-Khan, M. (2012). Telehealth for nursing homes: The utilization of specialist services for residential care. *Journal of Telemedicine and Telecare, 18*(3), 142-146. doi:10.1258/jtt.2012.sft105

Greenberg, M.E. (2009). A comprehensive model of the process of telephone nursing. *Journal of Advanced Nursing, 65*(12), 2621-2629.

Greenwood, A. (n.d.). *Value of nursing project: Phase 1.* Retrieved from https://healthimpact.org/wp-content/uploads/2016/03/Final-Product-VON_1-MAR-2016.pdf

Greving, J.P., Kaasjager, H.A., Vernooij, J.W., Hovens, M.M., Wierdsma, J., Grandjean, H.M., ... Visseren, F.L. (2015). Cost-effectiveness of a nurse-led Internet-based vascular risk factor management programme: Economic evaluation alongside a randomised controlled clinical trial. *BMJ Open, 5*(5). doi:10.1136/bmjopen-2014-007128

Gustafson, D., Wise, M., Bhattacharya, A., Pulvermacher, A., Shanovich, K., Phillips, B., & Kim, J. (2012). The effects of combining web-based ehealth with telephone nurse case management for pediatric asthma control: A randomized controlled trial. *Journal of Medical Internet Research, 14*(4). doi:10.2196/jmir.1964

Harvey, S., Peterkin, G., & Wootton, R. (2010). Eleven years of experience with low-bandwidth telemedicine in a nurse-led rural clinic in Scotland. *Journal of Telemedicine and Telecare, 16*(8), 417-421. doi:10.1258/jtt.2010.100310

Hughes, R. (2008). *Patient safety and quality: An evidence-based handbook for nurses.* Rockville, MD: Agency for Healthcare Research and Quality.

Institute of Medicine (IOM). (2010). *The future of nursing: Leading change, advancing health.* Washington, DC: National Academies Press.

Klasner, A.E., King, W.D., Crews, T.B., & Monroe, K.W. (2006). Accuracy and response time when clerks are used for telephone triage. *Clinical Pediatrics, 45*(3), 267-269.

Jerome, L.W., & Zaylor, C. (2000). Cyberspace: Creating a therapeutic environment for telehealth applications. *Professional Psychology: Research and Practice, 31*(5), 478-483.

Kiernan, T.J., & Demaerschalk, B.M. (2010). Nursing roles within a stroke telemedicine network. *Journal of Central Nervous System Disease, 2*, 1-7. doi:10.4137/jcnsd.s4284

Kimman, M., Dirksen, C., Voogd, A., Falger, P., Gijsen, B., Thuring, M., ... Boersma, L. (2011). Nurse-led telephone follow-up and an educational group programme after breast cancer treatment: Results of a 2×2 randomised controlled trial. *European Journal of Cancer, 47*(7), 1027-1036. doi:10.1016/j.ejca.2010.12.003

Lipstein, S.H., & Kellermann, A.L. (2016). Workforce for 21st-century health and health care. *JAMA, 316*(16), 1665.

Looman, W.S., Erickson, M.M., Garwick, A.W., Cady, R.G., Kelly, A., Pettey, C., & Finkelstein, S.M. (2012). Meaningful use of data in care coordination by the advanced practice RN. *CIN: Computers, Informatics, Nursing, 30*(12), 649-654. doi:10.1097/nxn.0b013e318266caf2

Lustig, T.A. (2012). *The role of telehealth in an evolving health care environment: Workshop summary.* Washington, DC: National Academies Press.

Marconi, G.P., Chang, T., Pham, P.K., Grajower, D.N., & Nager, A.L. (2014). Traditional nurse triage vs physician telepresence in a pediatric ED. *The American Journal of Emergency Medicine, 32*(4), 325-329. doi:10.1016/j.ajem.2013.12.032

Minatodani, D.E., Chao, P.J., & Berman, S.J. (2013). Home telehealth: Facilitators, barriers, and impact of nurse support among high-risk dialysis patients. *Telemedicine and e-Health, 19*(8), 573-578. doi:10.1089/tmj.2012.0201

Mollerup, A., Harboe, G., & Johansen, J. D. (2016). User evaluation of patient counselling, combining nurse consultation and eHealth in hand eczema. *Contact Dermatitis, 74*(4), 205-216. doi:10.1111/cod.12534

Mort, M., Roberts, C., Pols, J., Domenech, M., & Moser, I. (2013). Ethical implications of home telecare for older people: A framework derived from a multisited participative study. *Health Expectations, 18*(3), 438-449. doi:10.1111/hex.12109

Muir, K.W., Grubber, J., Mruthyunjaya, P., Mccant, F., & Bosworth, H.B. (2013). Progression of diabetic retinopathy in the hypertension intervention nurse telemedicine study. *JAMA Ophthalmology, 131*(7), 957. doi:10.1001/jamaophthalmol.2013.81

Nagel, D.A., Pomerleau, S.G., & Penner, J.L. (2012). Knowing, caring, and telehealth technology. *Journal of Holistic Nursing, 31*(2), 104-112. doi:10.1177/0898010112465357

Navratil-Strawn, J.L., Ozminkowski, R.J., & Hartley, S.K. (2014). An economic analysis of a nurse-led telephone triage service. *Journal of Telemedicine and Telecare, 20*(6), 330-338. doi:10.1177/1357633x14545430

Ovbiagele, B. (2015). Phone-based intervention under nurse guidance after stroke: Concept for lowering blood pressure after stroke in sub-saharan Africa. *Journal of Stroke and Cerebrovascular Diseases, 24*(1), 1-9. doi:10.1016/j.jstrokecerebrovasdis.2014.08.011

Palen, T.E., Price, D., Shetterly, S., & Wallace, K.B. (2012). Comparing virtual consults to traditional consults using an electronic health record: An observational case – control study. *BMC Medical Informatics and Decision Making, 12*(1).

Pols, J. (2010). The heart of the matter. About good nursing and telecare. *Health Care Analysis, 18*(4), 374-388. doi:10.1007/s10728-009-0140-1

Wolf, D.M., Anton, B.B., & Wenskovitch, J. (2014). Promoting health and safety virtually: Key recommendations for occupational health nurses. *Workplace Health & Safety, 62*(7), 307-307. doi:10.3928/21650799-20140617-06

Reierson, I., Solli, H., & Bjørk, I. T. (2015). Nursing students perspectives on telenursing in patient care after simulation. *Clinical Simulation in Nursing, 11*(4), 244-250. doi:10.1016/j.ecns.2015.02.003

Romero, Y.M., Angelo, M., & Gonzalez, L.A. (2012). Imaginative construction of care: The nursing professional experience in a remote care service. *Revista Latino-Americana de Enfermagem, 20*(4), 693-700. doi:10.1590/s0104-11692012000400009

Ruesch, C., Mossakowski, J., Forrest, J., Hayes, M., Jahrsdoerfer, M., Comeau, E., & Schmitt, B.D. (2008). Telephone triage liability: Protecting your patients and your practice from harm. *Advances in Pediatrics, 55*(1), 29-42.

Schmitt, B. D. (2016). *Pediatric telephone protocols: Office version* (15th ed.). Elk Grove Village, IL: American Academy of Pediatrics.

Schroeder, R. (2008). Defining virtual worlds and virtual environments. *Journal for Virtual Worlds Research, 1*(1).

Singleton, M. (2012). Using nursing expertise and telemedicine to increase nursing collaboration and improve patient outcomes. *Telemedicine and e-Health, 18*(8), 591-595.

Rutenberg, C. (2014). *Telephone triage program design supporting best practices.* Retrieved from http://www.nyscha.org/files/2014/handouts/TH-3.02%20Telephone%20Triage%20Program%20Design.pdf

Rutenberg, C. (2016). *Telephone triage program design and implementation in the clinic setting: Lessons learned in 20 tears of consulting.* Retrieved from http://www.prolibraries.com/aaacn/?select=session&sessionID=580

Ryu, S. (2012). Telemedicine: Opportunities and developments in member states: Report on the Second Global Survey on eHealth 2009 (Global Observatory for eHealth Series, Volume 2). *Healthcare Informatics Research, 18*(2), 153. doi:10.4258/hir.2012.18.2.153

Sanches, L.M., Alves, D.S., Lopes, M.H., & Novaes, M.A. (2012). The practice of telehealth by nurses: An experience in primary healthcare in Brazil. *Telemedicine and e-Health, 18*(9), 679-683. doi:10.1089/tmj.2012.0011

Segar, J., Rogers, A., Salisbury, C., & Thomas, C. (2013). Roles and identities in transition: Boundaries of work and inter-professional relationships at the interface between telehealth and primary care. *Health & Social Care in the Community, 21*(6), 606-613.

Sharvill, N.J. (2012). Daily contact with a nurse may be more important than high tech telecare. *BMJ, 344*, e875. doi:10.1136/bmj.e875

Totten, A.M., Womack, D.M., Eden, K.B., McDonagh, M.S., Griffin, J.C., Grusing, S., & Hersh, W.R. (2016). *Telehealth: Mapping the evidence for patient outcomes from systematic reviews.* Rockville, MD: Agency for Healthcare Research and Quality.

Tubaishat, A., & Habiballah, L. (2016). EHealth literacy among undergraduate nursing students. *Nurse Education Today, 42*, 47-52. doi:10.1016/j.nedt.2016.04.003

Tuxbury, J.S. (2013). The experience of presence among telehealth nurses. *Journal of Nursing Research, 21*(3), 155-161. doi:10.1097/jnr.0b013e3182a0b028

Wachter, D., Brillman, J., Lewis, J., & Sapien, R. (1999). Pediatric telephone triage protocols: Standardized decisionmaking or a false sense of security? *Annals of Emergency Medicine, 33*(4), 388-394

Wakefield, B.J., Scherubel, M., Ray, A., & Holman, J.E. (2013). Nursing interventions in a telemonitoring program. *Telemedicine and e-Health, 19*(3), 160-165.

Wentzel, J., Van Velsen, L., Van Limburg, M., De Jong, N., Karreman, J., Hendrix, R., & Van Gemert-Pijnen, J. (2014). Participatory eHealth development to support nurses in antimicrobial stewardship. *BMC Medical Informatics Decision Making.* Retrieved from https://bmcmedinformdecismak.biomedcentral.com/articles/10.1186/1472-6947-14-45

What is Machine Learning? (2018). *What is machine learning? A definition.* Retrieved from http://www.expertsystem.com/machine-learning-definition/

White, K.M., & O'Sullivan, A. (2012). *The essential guide to nursing practice: Applying ANAs scope and standards in practice and education.* Silver Spring, MD: American Nurses Association.

Xu, C., Jackson, M., Scuffham, P. A., Wootton, R., Simpson, P., Whitty, J., ... Wainwright, C. E. (2010). A randomized controlled trial of an interactive voice response telephone system and specialist nurse support for childhood asthma management. *Journal of Asthma, 47*(7), 768-773. doi:10.3109/02770903.2010.493966

Young, H., Miyamoto, S., Ward, D., Dharmar, M., Tang-Feldman, Y., & Berglund, L. (2014). Sustained effects of a nurse coaching intervention via telehealth to improve health behavior change in diabetes. *Telemedicine and e-Health, 20*(9), 828-834. doi:10.1089/tmj.2013.0326

Zahs, C.M., & Hagen, M.M. (2015). A day in the life of a telehealth nurse. *Home Healthcare Now, 33*(6), 342-343.